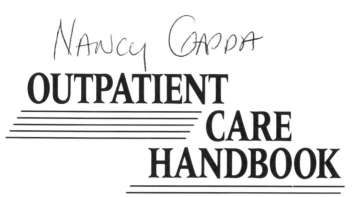

Nancy Gappa

OUTPATIENT
CARE
HANDBOOK

PETER A. GLASSMAN, M.Sc., M.D.

Clinical Instructor in General Internal Medicine
University of California at Los Angeles
Research Fellow in Primary Care
West Los Angeles Veterans Affairs Medical Center
Los Angeles, California

DANIEL GARCIA, M.D.

Assistant Professor of Medicine
University of California at Los Angeles
Los Angeles, California
Staff Internist
Sepulveda Veterans Affairs Medical Center
Sepulveda, California

JUDITH P. DELAFIELD, Ph.D., M.D.

Assistant Professor of Medicine
University of California at Los Angeles
Director of General Medical Clinics
West Los Angeles Veterans Affairs Medical Center
Los Angeles, California

HANLEY & BELFUS, INC./Philadelphia
MOSBY–YEAR BOOK, INC./St. Louis • Baltimore • Boston
Chicago • London • Philadelphia • Sydney • Toronto

Publisher: HANLEY & BELFUS, INC.
                  210 South 13th Street
                  Philadelphia, PA 19107
                  (215) 546-7293

North American and worldwide sales and distribution:

                  MOSBY-YEAR BOOK, INC.
                  11830 Westline Industrial Drive
                  St. Louis, MO 63146

In Canada: THE C.V. MOSBY COMPANY
                  5240 Finch Avenue East
                  Unit 1
                  Scarborough, Ontario M1S 4P2

OUTPATIENT CARE HANDBOOK   ISBN 1-56053-057-X

The authors and publisher have taken care to ensure that the patient
care recommended herein, including choice of drugs and drug dosages,
is in accord with the accepted standards and practice at the time of
publication. However, because research and regulation constantly
change clinical standards, the reader is urged to check the product
information sheet included in the package of each drug, which includes
recommended doses, warnings, and contraindications. This is particularly
important with new or infrequently used drugs.

Last digit is the print number: 9   8   7   6   5   4   3   2   1

CONTENTS

Part VI
PRIMARY CARE FOR ADULTS

Contents

Part VII
MEDICAL DECISION-MAKING

Part VIII
APPENDICES

Part IX
INDEX OF CONSENSUSES

SUBJECT INDEX

PREFACE

"Practicing medicine . . . until we get it right"
Firesign Theater

This handbook is a concise guide to the evaluation and management of common problems encountered in outpatient general internal medicine. Each chapter contains—in outline form—general principles, relevant facts, and essentials of the medical history and physical examination. The initial and secondary investigations needed for evaluating each medical problem are listed, along with an approach to each problem's management. The book gives additional information regarding referrals to specialists, and it also provides the reader with important screening tools and useful equations.

The protocols presented in this book are, as often as possible, derived from guidelines detailed in consensus papers. The organizations writing such guidelines include nationally recognized medical organizations such as the American College of Physicians (ACP), the American Medical Association (AMA) and its affiliates, the Centers for Disease Control (CDC), the National Institutes of Health (NIH), the RAND Corporation, and the United States Preventive Services Task Force. This information was supplemented with clinical reviews, randomized control trials, editorials, and personal experience when consensuses were lacking or had insufficient detail.

We wrote this book so that physicians will have, in one place, a way to rapidly access some of the widely dispersed medical literature that practitioners are so often expected to know, understand, and use. We recognize that no single set of recommendations will satisfy all physicians, but our hope is that interested readers will review and critique our work, especially as new information and clinical guidelines become available. Practitioners must, in the final analysis, use their clinical sense for guidance. Our goal is to provide practitioners with an effective and efficient tool to assist in clinical decision-making.

ACKNOWLEDGMENTS

We gratefully acknowledge the support and advice of our reviewers, who graciously contributed their time and help: Joel Braslow MD, PhD, Bruce Chernof, MD, Stanley Cohen MD, Susan Cook NP, Jeff Etchason MD, Jacob Fleischman MD, Ann Flitcraft MD, Diedre Gifford MD, David Gordon MD, Steven Hayashi MD, Jerome Hershman MD, Bernie Klein MD, Jill Klessig MD, Paul Lee MD, Alan Lichtenstein MD, Mark Litwin MD, Jerry Markowitz MD, Christopher

Ng MD, Bonnie Olson MD, Daniel Rodriguez MD, Nate Ross MD, Cydney Stewart MD, Aida Vega MD, Monica Wells PharmD, and Michael Wilkes MD, MPH.

We also would like to thank the following for their assistance in helping to bring the book to fruition: Howard Bennett, MD, Samuel A. Bozzette, MD, Raymond Hall, DC, Mrs. Sarah Lesser, Marlene Nishimoto, Joy Williams, and the reference librarians at the West Los Angeles Veterans Affairs Medical Center. And very special thanks to Lisa Hoffman, now Glassman.

Peter A. Glassman, M.Sc., M.D.
Daniel Garcia, M.D.
Judith P. Delafield, Ph.D., M.D.

PART I
INTRODUCTION

Attributes of an Internist

I. **Definition of the General Internist**

A general internist is defined by the American Board of Internal Medicine (ABIM) as "a physician who provides scientifically based, empathic care for the nonsurgical illnesses of adolescents and adults"

II. **General Principles**

A. **Attributes of a general internist**
1. Commitment and dedication to the patient
2. Stable, supportive and caring relationship with the patient
3. Making time, when needed, for the patient
4. Maintaining professional skills and technical prowess
5. Personal interest in patient welfare
6. Providing medical consultations with specialist physicians
7. Competent basic emergency and critical care
8. Competent ambulatory and in-patient care for persons with simple or complex medical problems
9. Advocacy for the patient

B. **Medical residency** should attempt to engender in each resident
1. Proficiency in gathering data
2. Ability to use clinical skills for diagnosis and management
3. Understanding of the pathogenesis of disease
4. Desire for continuous improvement through education and self-study
5. Ability to use new knowledge and new technologies to provide effective care for patients
6. Humanitarian attitude in both action and thought toward those in need of assistance

Reference

The above quote and attributes are taken or modified from: Council on General Internal Medicine of the American Board of Internal Medicine: Attributes of the general internist and recommendations for training. Am Rev Respir Dis 134:371, 1986.

Medical Ethics

I. **General Principles: Basic Concepts that Govern Medical Ethics**

   A. **Autonomy:** the right of patient choice
   1. Failure to respect a rational and competent individual's decision may constitute assault
   2. A psychiatric consultation to prove competency is unnecessary if, by clinical evaluation, the patient is competent

   B. **Beneficence:** "being of benefit to the patient," which engenders in the physician a desire to be a patient's advocate for the best available care

   C. **Nonmalfeasance:** the tenet of DO NO HARM

   D. **Informed consent:** an agreement to treat based on the patient's understanding of the risks and benefits that "a reasonable person" would want to know

   E. **Fiduciary trust:** the keeping of patient confidentiality

II. **Specific Issues**

   A. **The relationship of caring**
   1. A physician and patient enter into a mutual contract for care
   2. A physician cannot discriminate against any race, creed, color, national origin, gender, sexual preference, or individual characteristic
   3. A physician may refuse to initiate treatment unless
      a. No other physician is available
      b. A patient is in need of emergency care
   4. A physician can discontinue providing care if:
      a. The patient is notified and agrees
      b. The patient suffers no harm by transfer of care to another provider
      c. Continuity of care is ensured

   B. **The risk of caring**
   1. A physician cannot refuse to treat an individual because of real or perceived risk (e.g., from HIV) to him or herself
      a. This may not apply when the patient threatens the physician with physical harm

   C. **Finances and contractual obligations**
   1. The physician is responsible for ensuring appropriate care to a patient once the physician and patient have entered into an established relationship

   D. **Confidentiality**
   1. The physician must maintain confidentiality unless
      a. The release of information is required by law
      b. The information is necessary to save another person from physical harm

E. **The medical record**
1. Belongs to the physician/institution (laws vary by state)
2. Patients may not be denied knowledge of the contents
3. Individual states have laws governing the patient's right of direct access to the chart
4. A physician must abide by a patient's written request to transfer documents to a third party

F. **Consent**
1. The physician must inform the patient and/or patient's surrogate of
    a. Diagnosis and general medical condition
    b. Diagnostic procedures and treatment
    c. Risks of the condition, diagnostics, and treatment
    d. Alternative diagnostic procedures and treatments
2. It is the patient's or surrogate's ethical and legal right to consent to or refuse any procedure
    a. Unless a court rules otherwise
3. It is the physician's obligation to explain, in terms the patient (surrogate) can understand, the risks and benefits of any proposed procedure or treatment plan

G. **Consultation**
1. It may be appropriate to request a consultation if
    a. Proper diagnosis or medical care necessitates input from another provider
    b. The patient or proxy decision-maker requests a consultation
2. It is unethical to collude with another provider for purposes of monetary gain

H. **Conflicts of interest**
1. Patient welfare always takes precedence over fiscal loss or gain to the physician
2. Receiving "kickback" money for referrals, use of a facility, procedure, or medication is unethical

I. **Competent patients and medical care**
1. A competent patient, well informed of diagnosis, risks, and prognosis, may refuse procedures, care, therapy, resuscitative measures, and other life-sustaining treatment(s)
2. Only the patient (or state/federal law) can countermand his or her decision(s) unless the patient is declared incompetent by a court of law
3. A patient's decision is discussed with family and friends only with permission from the patient
4. A patient's decision(s) should be documented and updated periodically

J. **Incompetent patients and decision-making**
1. A proxy decision-maker must be legally and morally responsible for the incompetent patient's welfare
2. The concept of "substituted judgment" refers to ascertaining what the patient would have wanted in a given situation

3. Advanced directives or living wills are helpful but are not, in most states, legally binding
   a. Directives should be updated periodically
4. The physician should attempt to document a patient's wishes while the patient is competent

K. Other considerations

1. Physicians who object to contraception or abortion or other medical practices should ensure that a patient has the option of seeking advice from a qualified practitioner who does not hold such beliefs

III. Improper or Unethical Behaviors

A. It is immoral, unethical, and/or illegal to
   1. Participate in **nonscientific conduct or therapeutics**, including the use of "secret remedies"
   2. Degrade or disparage, without evidence of wrongdoing, another physician or his/her services
   3. Avoid reporting known fraudulent activity by or misconduct of another physician
   4. Avoid the reporting of impaired physicians (e.g., alcoholism, psychiatric disease) to the relevant authorities (i.e., chief resident, hospital committee, state agency)
   5. Engage in active euthanasia (mercy killing, assisted suicide)
   6. Participate in torture

Reference

The above section is modified from: American College of Physicians: American College of Physicians Ethics Manual, Parts I and II. Ann Intern Med 111:245–252, 327–335, 1989.

PART II
ADOLESCENT MEDICINE

I. General Principles
A. Areas of specific concern in adolescent medicine
1. Growth and development
2. Substance abuse
3. Violence and accidents
4. Eating disorders
5. Sexually transmitted diseases, including HIV/AIDS

B. Common problems
1. Obesity affects 5–25% of adolescents
2. Physical handicaps affect about 10% of <18-year-olds
3. Around 50% of high school seniors have used marijuana
4. Alcohol-related problems often occur in families where parent(s) is (are) heavy drinker(s) or where they abstain
5. Sexual, physical, or mental abuse may occur at any time
6. Once puberty is reached, adolescents grow through about one Tanner stage per year

II. Diagnostics
A. Medical history
1. Family history: hypertension, coronary artery disease, adult-onset diabetes mellitus
2. Diethylstilbestrol exposure in utero
3. Childhood disease and immunization status
4. Medical problems
5. Mental health, including suicide risk (ideation and/or attempts) and sexual and/or physical abuse
6. Reproductive history, sexual habits, contraceptive use
7. Relationships: conflicts with family, peers
8. School and/or work performance
9. Hobbies and social activities
10. Sports: injuries, use of anabolic steroids
11. Substance use: tobacco, drugs, alcohol
12. Dental and eye exams
13. Knowledge of HIV/AIDS and safe sex
14. Diet and exercise habits
15. Driving habits
    a. Use of seat belts
    b. Driving while under the influence of alcohol or drugs

B. Examination
1. BP measurement
2. Height and weight (see Appendix 1, p. 279)
3. Sexual development (see Appendix 2, p. 281)
4. Visual acuity (at least once during adolescence)

      5. Full physical (at least once during adolescence)
      6. Back exam for scoliosis
      7. Pelvic exam with Pap smear (yearly), if sexually active

  C. **Laboratory data**
     1. **Initial investigations**
        a. Cholesterol screening should begin by age 20
           i. Early screening with **fasting lipoprotein analysis** is recommended for adolescents whose parents or grandparents have documented atherosclerosis (e.g., MI, PVD, angina, CVA, sudden cardiac death) at or before age 55
           ii. Early screening with **nonfasting total cholesterol** is recommended for adolescents with a parent who has total cholesterol of 240 mg/dl or higher and for adolescents with unknown family history
           iii. Early screening with **nonfasting total cholesterol** may be considered for adolescents who may have increased risk of CHD (without a family history of such), for instance, those with hypertension, obesity, and smoking history
     2. **For selected asymptomatic patients,** consider screening with
        a. Urinalysis
        b. Cultures of vaginal secretions for asymptomatic STDs in sexually active adolescents
        c. Complete blood count
           i. In young women, especially if recent immigrant and/or from disadvantaged socioeconomic background
        d. Sickle cell preparations
        e. HIV antibody tests for those in high-risk categories
        f. Hepatitis B antibody tests for those in high-risk groups

III. **Management**

  A. **General approach**: discussion with each individual should include
     1. Methods of safe sex and contraception, including how HIV is transmitted
     2. Advice on periodic dental care and eye exams
     3. Danger of high-risk behaviors
        a. Drinking alcohol and driving
        b. Substance use
        c. Gang activities
        d. Gun and knife use
     4. Ensuring immunizations are up to date
        a. Some patients may need primary series, whereas most will need, at some time, booster doses of certain vaccinations
        b. Risk groups (e.g., homosexuals, IV drug users) may need hepatitis B vaccination
     5. Other dangerous driving habits
        a. Racing cars
        b. Attention-seeking behavior
        c. Tension-releasing driving (fast and reckless)

B. **For specific patients**
  1. **General screening**
     a. For normotensive patients (systolic BP <140 mmHg and diastolic BP <90 mmHg)
        i. Recheck BP within 2 yr
     b. For sexually active adolescent women
        i. Yearly Pap smear and cultures of vaginal secretions
     c. For patients 20 yr and older
        i. Advise on low saturated fat diet and reducing other cardiac rick factors (e.g., smoking)
        ii. For cholesterol <200 mg/dl, recheck in 5 yr
        iii. For cholesterol 200 mg/dl or greater, see chapter on "Cholesterol and Lipids" for details
     d. For adolescents under age 20
        i. Advise on low saturated fat diet and reducing other cardiac risk factors (e.g., smoking)
        ii. For total cholesterol ≤170 mg/dl, recheck in 5 yr
        iii. For total cholesterol between 170 and 199 mg/dl, repeat total cholesterol and average with first measurement. If average is ≤170 mg/dl, recheck total cholesterol in 5 yr. If repeat total cholesterol is >170 mg/dl, do lipoprotein analysis (TC, LDL, HDL, triglycerides)
        iv. If total cholesterol is ≥200 mg/dl, do fasting lipoprotein analysis
     e. Management of fasting lipoprotein analysis results
        i. Repeat initial test and average with previous measurement for more accurate LDL level
        ii. For LDL <110 mg/dl, repeat lipoprotein analysis within 5 yr
        iii. For LDL between 110 and 129 mg/dl,
           • Give risk factor advice
           • Put on step one diet
           • Recheck lipoprotein analysis within 1 yr
        iv. For LDL ≥130 mg/dl
           • Evaluate for secondary causes and familial disorders (screen family members)
           • Reduce LDL to at least <130 mg/dl (ideally <110 mg/dl) by using step one and step two diets, as needed
           • Recheck LDL after 6 wk on step one diet; if still ≥130 mg/dl, reinstruct on step one diet and recheck LDL after 3 mo; if still ≥130 mg/dl, go to step two diet and recheck after 3 mo
           • If minimal goal not achieved after above, consider drug therapy (discuss with specialist in adolescent medicine) and/or cholesterol and lipids
     d. Dietary advice
        i. Step one diet
           • Total fat, <30% of total calories
           • Saturated fats, <10% of total calories

- Polyunsaturated fats, up to 10% of total calories
- Monounsaturated fats, remaining total fat calories
- Cholesterol <300 mg/d
- Carbohydrates, about 55% of total calories
- Protein, about 15–20% total calories
- Calories, as necessary for normal growth pattern

  ii. Step two diet

    (a) Same as step one diet except that saturated fats should be <7% of total calories and cholesterol should be <200 mg/d

3. If **growth or developmental deficit is suspected**
   a. Take family history for heights in each parent
   b. Review, if data available, growth over time
   c. Evaluate secondary sexual development
   d. Differential should include
      i. Eating disorder
      ii. Delayed puberty (if no pubertal development by age 14)
      iii. Hypothalamic–pituitary–gonadal disease
      iv. Systemic diseases
         (a) Hypothyroidism
         (b) Inflammatory bowel disease
         (c) Renal dysfunction
         (d) Anemia
   e. Assess psychosocial aspects of short stature
4. If **eating disorder is suspected**
   a. See chapter on "Eating Disorders" for details of diagnosis and management
5. If **substance or alcohol abuse is suspected,** assess
   a. Quantity and type used
   b. Duration and patterns of use
   c. Dependency status
      i. Experimentation
      ii. Casual/social use
      iii. Regular use with "need" for alcohol/drug
   d. Psychosocial aspects of drug use
      i. Family/peer relationships
      ii. School/work performance and attendance
      iii. Family/peer substance or alcohol use
      iv. Legal difficulties
   e. General medical problems associated with drug(s)

References

1. American College of Physicians: Health care needs of the adolescent. Ann Intern Med 110:930–935, 1989.
2. D'Angelo, Farrow J: Clinical problems in adolescent medicine. J Gen Intern Med 4:64–73, 1989.
3. National Cholesterol Education Program. Highlights of the Report of the Expert Panel on Blood Cholesterol Levels in Children and Adolescents. National Institutes of Health. Publication No. 91-2731. September 1991.

PART III
OCCUPATIONAL AND ENVIRONMENTAL MEDICINE

General Approach and the Occupational History

"There is virtually no major chronic disease to which environmental factors do not contribute, either directly or indirectly."
—*Surgeon General's Report on Health Promotion, 1979*

I. **General Principles**

A. **Workers' compensation and liability litigation**
1. Only a 50% chance that a condition is related to occupation may be needed
2. A court may assign a percent liability that is significantly lower than 50%

B. **Basic goals** of occupational/environmental assessment
1. Identify any major risks
2. Interpret risks for a particular patient
3. Take steps to reduce the risks

C. **Major risks**
1. **Chemical** hazards
   a. Lead, cadmium, mercury
   b. Synthetic fibers
      i. Asbestos
   c. Airborne particles
      i. Wood dust
   d. Pesticides
      i. Organophosphates and other types of pesticides
   e. Alloys
   f. Solvents
2. **Environmental** hazards
   a. Air pollution
   b. Ultraviolet radiation
   c. Cold household temperatures
   d. Toxic waste
   e. Radon
   f. Excessive noise
   g. Vibration
3. **Biologic** hazards
   a. Infectious diseases
   b. Allergens

D. **Jobs at risk:** See Appendix 3, p. 282

II. **Diagnostics**

    A. **Occupational history form**: See Appendix 4, p 286

III. **Management**

    A. **General approach**
1. Counsel on risks of exposure(s) and concurrent risks (e.g., smoking and asbestosis)
2. Advise removal from risk factor and if necessary advise patient to change jobs if risk is work-related
3. Contact the employer's environmental safety officer
4. Contact local Occupational Safety and Health Administration (OSHA) in phone book under Labor Department
5. Contact National Institute of Occupational Safety and Health (NIOSH)
    NIOSH
    ATTN: Information Retrieval and Analysis Section
    4676 Columbia Parkway
    Cincinnati, OH 45226
    Telephone 1-800-356-4674
6. Contact the local Department of Health for referral to the local center for disease control
7. Other databases
    a. The National Library of Medicine
        i. TOXLINE (on computer)
        ii. Hazardous Substances Data Bank
    b. National Cancer Institute
        i. Chemical Carcinogenesis Research Information System
    c. Centers for Disease Control
        i. Center for Environmental Health and Injury Control

    B. **Specific measures** depend on type of disease
1. See chapters on "Asbestosis" and "Occupational Asthma" for details on diagnosis and management of these common occupational diseases

    C. **Referral** to an Occupational Disease Specialist
1. Referral is often prudent and helpful when evaluation(s) suggests an occupational disease

Reference

For further information and bibliography consult: American College of Physicians. Occupational and environmental medicine: The internist's role. Ann Intern Med 113:974–982, 1990.

Asbestosis: Diagnostic Evaluation

I. **Definition**

Asbestos refers to a set of hydrated silicate fibers that, when inhaled in sufficient quantity, can produce interstitial fibrosis of the pulmonary parenchyma (asbestosis) and/or pleural abnormalities

II. **General Principles**
  A. An estimated 27,500,000 persons may have had exposure to asbestos from the end of WWII to 1979
  B. Severe interstitial fibrosis with asbestos bodies (with or without a history of exposure) is considered diagnostic for asbestosis
  C. Asbestos inhalation does not always lead to asbestosis
  D. The risk of asbestosis rises with duration and quantity of exposure
  E. Diagnosis is usually determined clinically by
    1. Exposure history
    2. Interval from exposure to disease
    3. Pulmonary function tests
    4. CXR abnormalities
  F. Diagnosis rarely requires a lung biopsy

III. **Lung Abnormalities Seen with Asbestosis**
  A. **Benign pleural abnormalities**
    1. Pleural plaques
      a. Discrete, diffuse or nodular, raised
      b. Usually on posterolateral, lower pleura, but not at costophrenic angles
    2. Pleural thickening
      a. Pleural fibrosis that may impair pulmonary function
    3. Pleural effusion
      a. Early manifestation of asbestos exposure
      b. Can occur within several years after exposure
      c. May occur/recur unilaterally or bilaterally
  B. **Benign parenchymal fibrosis**
    1. Often starts at basal area and extends toward the apices
    2. Ranges from diffuse fibrosis to honeycombing
    3. Can severely restrict lung function
  C. **Other asbestos-related diseases**
    1. Malignant mesothelioma
      a. Usually occurs >25 yr after exposure
      b. Diagnosis is often made by pleural biopsy
    2. Bronchogenic carcinomas
      a. Significant rise in risk when asbestosis combined with cigarette smoking

IV. **Diagnostics**

  A. **History**
1. Occupational history
2. Estimated amount of time exposed
3. Type of asbestos, if known
4. Dyspnea
5. Pleuritic chest pain
6. Presence of symptoms of other systemic disease that may cause fibrosis
   a. Other occupational toxins
      i. Noxious gases
      ii. Beryllium
      iii. Silicosis
   b. Drugs
      i. Bleomycin and other chemotherapeutic agents
   c. Autoimmune disease
   d. Sarcoid

  B. **Examination**
1. Respiratory rate
2. Fingernail clubbing
3. Basal paninspiratory crepitations

  C. **Laboratory data**
1. Initial investigations
   a. Chest x-ray
      i. May have one or a combination of the following
         (a) Pleural plaques
         (b) Pleural thickening
         (c) Irregular interstitial fibrosis
         (d) Small, irregular opacifications: fine, medium, or coarse
   b. Pulmonary function tests
      i. Decreased vital capacity and diffusing capacity (DLCO)
      ii. Normal or near normal FEV/FVC (restrictive picture)
      iii. Reduced lung volumes
   c. Electrocardiogram
      i. Right ventricular hypertrophy or cor pulmonale as indicated by right atrial abnormality "p pulmonale"
2. Further evaluation
   a. CT scan of lungs can show more plaques than a CXR
   b. Lung biopsy
      i. This is rarely done but should be considered if the diagnosis is unable to be made by evaluations above
      ii. Patients should be evaluated by a pulmonologist or occupational disease specialist before this test is considered

V. Management

A. Asbestosis is an insidious disease with no effective therapy; patients need
  1. Supportive care for lung disease
  2. Advice on stopping cigarettes
  3. Long-term follow-up and monitoring
  4. Advice on seeking compensation for illness
B. General information can also be obtained from
  1. NIOSH
  2. State and/or local regulatory agencies

VI. Referral to a Pulmonary or Occupational Disease Specialist

A. Uncertainty of diagnosis
B. Evaluation after preliminary tests
C. Suspicion of additional lung disease (e.g., carcinoma or mesothelioma)

Reference

American Thoracic Society: The diagnosis of nonmalignant diseases related to asbestos. Am Rev Respir Dis 134:363–368, 1986.

Occupational Asthma: Diagnosis and Management

I. Definition

Airway hyperresponsiveness triggered by an allergen found in the workplace

II. General Principles

A. The prevalence of occupational asthma may range from 5–20% in certain industries
B. Over 200 substances are known to cause bronchospasm
C. **Persons at risk** include those who work with
  1. Animals: often small mammals (rats, mice, rabbits)
  2. Grain (or flour) dust
  3. Textiles: cotton, flax, hemp, jute
  4. Irritant gases or fumes: plastic manufacturing, toxic wastes
  5. Organophosphates: agricultural insecticides
  6. Isocyanates
  7. Wood dust: western red cedar, redwood, oak
  8. Biologic enzymes: trypsin, pancreatin, pepsin
  9. Metals: nickel, platinum, cobalt

III. **Diagnostics**

    A. **History**

        1. Occupational history

            a. Exposures to toxins, noxious gases, and fumes

        2. Duration of symptoms

        3. Relationship of symptoms to work (often delayed until night)

        4. Alleviation of symptoms by absence from work (e.g., vacations, weekends) with recurrence after return to work

        5. Presence of allergic symptoms (rhinitis, itchy eyes)

        6. Presence of asthma in other workers

        7. Cigarette smoking

        8. Other precipitants of asthma

    B. **Examination**

        1. Respiratory exam as per evaluation of asthma

        2. Presence of signs of allergy

            a. Conjunctivitis and blepharitis

            b. Dermatitis

    C. **Laboratory data**

        1. Peak flows at work and at home

            a. Take 3 readings every 2 hr throughout the day

                i. Keep written record for 1 wk **while at work**

                ii. Then record for 10 d **while off work**

                iii. Follow with record of **2 wk at work**

                iv. Plot differences over time

            b. Keep all medications stable during trial

                i. Can record readings t.i.d. if patient unable or unwilling to do so every 2 hr

        2. Pre- and post-work spirometric tests (peak flows)

            a. Sensitivity is relatively low

            b. Occupational asthma should not be excluded if test unhelpful

        3. Skin tests

            a. Some allergens can be tested for by skin patches (e.g., animal products, flour)

            b. Refer to allergist/immunologist for skin testing when specific allergen(s) are suspected in causing asthma

        4. Serologic tests

            a. RAST technique may help identify specific IgE antibodies

                i. Consult allergist/immunologist for details

        5. Bronchial provocation tests

            a. For specialist evaluation only

IV. **Management**

    A. Once work-related asthma is diagnosed, **remove worker from exposure**

        1. If worker refuses or cannot be moved

       a. Advise use of dust masks or respirators
       b. Monitor lung function periodically
       c. Treat asthma as per usual methods
          i. Beta agonists
         ii. Corticosteroids: oral/inhaled if needed
        iii. Theophylline derivatives
        iv. Cromolyn: if allergic symptoms present
         v. Anticholinergics: ipratropium bromide
       d. See chapter on "Asthma" for details regarding medications

B. It is advisable to **notify the state health department** because other workers may also have symptoms
C. If company refuses to move worker, consider contacting
   1. Patient's union liaison
   2. State health department
   3. Workers' Compensation Board
   4. NIOSH
D. Advise patient to stop smoking cigarettes

V. **Referral to Occupational Medicine Specialist or Pulmonologist for**
A. Uncertainty of diagnosis or management
B. Special diagnostic tests (also to dermatologist or allergist for skin and/or serologic tests)
C. Asthma recalcitrant to treatment or associated with concurrent lung disease
D. Follow-up and/or monitoring of disease
E. Severe recurrent asthma

References

1. Bardana EJ Jr, Montanaro A, O'Hollaren MT (eds): Occupational Asthma. Philadelphia, Hanley & Belfus, 1992.
2. Chan-Yeung M, Lam S: Occupational asthma. Am Rev Respir Dis 133:686–703, 1986.
3. Editorial: Asthma and work: How do you diagnose the association? Chest 100:1481–1482, 1991.

PART IV
PREVENTIVE CARE

General Approach and Recommendations for Adults

I. **General Principles**

   A. A number of organizations have developed recommendations for screening asymptomatic populations
   B. The recommendations offer similar perspectives but differ on some screening guidelines
   C. The recommendations below are based primarily on those given by the American College of Physicians
   D. Clinicians should consider those suggested by
      1. Canadian Task Force on Periodic Health Examination
      2. United States Preventive Services Task Force
      3. American Cancer Society
   E. Recommendations should be based on medical literature that discusses
      1. Population statistics: prevalence and incidence within general and specified populations
      2. Decision analysis of test results when applied to asymptomatic populations
      3. Explicit criteria for the screening program(s)
      4. Clinical significance of an intervention

II. **Recommendations**

   A. The following are for **asymptomatic adults without risk factors** for specific diseases
      1. For asymptomatic male adults
         a. Blood pressure every 2 yr if normotensive
         b. Cholesterol (nonfasting), starting by age 20 and continuing to age 70
            i. Remeasure every 5 yr if <200 mg/dl
            ii. For levels 200 mg/dl and above, see chapter on "Cholesterol and Lipids"
         c. Stool for occult blood every year after age 50
            i. Some guidelines recommend doing so after age 40
         d. Sigmoidoscopy: once every 3–5 yr, beginning at age 50
         e. Vaccination status (see chapter on "Immunizations" for details)
         f. Counseling (repeated as necessary)

          i. Safe sex and STD's
         ii. Exercise for health and bone strength
      iii. Nutrition: balanced diet, low fat
      iv. Injury prevention
       v. Addictions
      vi. Dental hygiene

2. For asymptomatic female adults
   a. Blood pressure every 2 yr if normotensive
   b. Cholesterol (nonfasting), starting by age 20 and continuing to age 70
      i. Remeasure every 5 yr if <200 mg/dl
      ii. For levels 200 mg/dl and above, see chapter on "Cholesterol and Lipids"
   c. Breast exam by a physician every year after age 35
   d. Pap smear: once a year after beginning sexual activity for the first 3 yr; if normal, then once every 3 yr until age 65
      i. Discontinue at 65 if previous smears × 3 have been normal
      ii. Some guidelines recommend continuing periodic Pap smear past age 65
   e. Stool for occult blood every year after age 50
      i. Some guidelines recommend doing so after age 40
   f. Sigmoidoscopy every 3–5 yr after age 50
   g. Mammography every year after age 50
      i. Guidelines differ on when to begin mammography
         (a) See chapter on "Breast Lesions" for details
   h. Vaccination status (see chapter on "Immunizations" for details)
   i. Counseling (repeated as necessary)
      i. Safe sex and STD's
      ii. Exercise for health and bone strength
      iii. Nutrition: balanced diet, low fat
      iv. Injury prevention
      v. Addictions
      vi. Dental hygiene
      vii. Osteoporosis prophylaxis (see chapter on "Osteoporosis" for details)

B. **Optional evaluations** in the asymptomatic patient
   1. Full physical exam, including oral exam, skin exam, testicular or pelvic exam, once every 1–3 yr
   2. Digital exam yearly after age 50 for prostate cancer
   3. Weight: yearly
   4. Self breast exam beginning in early adulthood
   5. Routine inquiry regarding functional status in elderly
   6. Screening for cognitive impairment in persons at risk (e.g., MMSE)
   7. Depression: maintain high index of suspicion

8. Vision
    a. Consider Snellen chart as general screen
        i. Periodic ophthalmologic consult
            • Especially in those over 65 (for glaucoma)
9. Hearing evaluation (otoscopic examination and/or audiometry)
    a. In the elderly
    b. If occupational or recreational history indicates regular exposure to loud noises
    c. History of hearing loss
10. **Optional laboratory studies** in asymptomatic individuals
    a. Creatinine: every 3–5 yr
    b. Urinalysis: every 3–5 yr
C. Further investigations for laboratory data on **asymptomatic persons in certain risk groups**
    1. HIV serology for members of any high-risk group
    2. Syphilis (VDRL, RPR) every 3–5 yr for
        a. HIV-infected persons
        b. History of previous infection
        c. Living in area of high prevalence
    3. Hemoglobin or hematocrit for
        a. Institutionalized elderly
        b. Recent immigrant, especially if from low socioeconomic group
        c. Menstruating women
    4. Thyroid studies (FT4 or FTI and TSH) for
        a. Patients >50 y/o with general symptoms that could be caused by thyroid dysfunction
        b. History of radiation exposure to neck
    5. Tuberculin testing (e.g., PPD)
        a. If exposure history at home
        b. If in community with high prevalence
        c. If HIV positive (yearly)
        d. Consider in alcoholics or persons with silicosis, gastrectomy or immunosuppression
        e. Consider in those who are recent immigrants or who live in high prevalence areas
    6. Electrocardiogram may be appropriate if
        a. Patient has one or more cardiac risk factors
        b. Patient is sedentary and >40 y/o and wants to start vigorous exercise program
    7. Bone mineral content
        a. Refer to chapter on "Osteoporosis" for details

References

1. Frontiers in disease prevention. J Gen Intern Med 5(5)(Suppl), 1990.
2. Guide to Clinical Preventative Services: An Assessment of the Effectiveness of 169 Interventions. Report of the U.S. Preventative Services Task Force. Baltimore, Williams & Wilkins, 1989.

3. Hayward RS, et al: Preventive care guidelines. Ann Intern Med 114:758–783, 1991.
4. Summary of Current Guidelines for the Cancer-Related Checkup. American Cancer Society, 1988.

Immunizations

I. General Principles

A. Most adults have completed their primary series of vaccinations and need only booster immunizations

B. In pregnant women it is generally advisable to delay needed vaccinations until the second or third trimester

C. In immunosuppressed persons, live viruses, BCG, and oral polio vaccine should not be used

   1. Short-term (<2 wk) corticosteroid treatment is not considered immunosuppressive

D. HIV-infected persons

   1. May receive MMR when indicated

      a. Physicians should discuss immunization with an ID specialist prior to administration

   2. May receive, when indicated, Td, enhanced-potency inactivated poliovirus (eIPV), pneumococcal, influenza, and hepatitis B vaccines

E. For information on vaccinations for travelers, see chapter on "Advice to Travelers"

II. Recommendations for Vaccine Use

A. Tetanus and diphtheria (Td) toxoids

   1. General considerations

      a. Efficacy of diphtheria toxoid series is at least 85%

      b. Efficacy of tetanus toxoid series is nearly 100%

   2. Primary series is 3 inoculations with doses 1 and 2 given 4 wk apart and dose 3 given 6–12 mo after dose 2

   3. Booster inoculations of tetanus toxoid are given every 10 yr

   4. Special considerations

      a. Booster dose is considered appropriate in patients with an unclean, penetrating wound and no tetanus inoculation within past 5 yr

      b. Patients with unknown history or no known history of Td series and an unclean, penetrating wound, should

         i. Be given tetanus immune globulin (TIG)

         ii. Have primary series begun and completed as per above protocol

      c. Previous neurologic or severe hypersensitivity reactions to tetanus toxoid are contraindications to further boosters

  d. Patients who have had Arthus-type reactions to tetanus toxoid can receive vaccine at 10-yr intervals but should not receive boosters more frequently

B. **Measles, mumps, and rubella (MMR)** (live viruses)
 1. Measles
  a. General considerations
   i. Efficacy of primary series is at least 95%
   ii. Adults born before 1957 are considered immune
   iii. Immunization should be given to
    (a) Adults born after 1956 without
     • Documentation of primary series on or after first birthday, or
     • History of physician-diagnosed measles, or
     • Serologic evidence of immunity
    (b) Those given inactivated measles vaccine (administered from 1963–1967)
  b. Primary series is 2 doses with both given 1 mo of each other
  c. Booster dose should be given if person has had only single inoculation in childhood and
   i. Exposure to measles is likely during an ongoing epidemic
   ii. He/she is traveling to endemic area
   iii. He/she is a health care worker
  d. Special considerations
   i. Vaccination should not be given to
    • Immunocompromised persons, except HIV-infected individuals (see General Principles above)
    • Pregnant women
    • Patients with egg allergy
   ii. Vaccine should not be given at the same time as immunoglobulin
 2. Mumps
  a. General considerations
   i. Efficacy of vaccine is estimated at 75–95%
   ii. Immunization should be given to adults born after 1956 with no history of having had mumps or a single mumps vaccination
  b. Primary series is single dose
  c. Booster dose is not necessary, but it is given coincidentally with second inoculation for measles
  d. Special considerations
   i. Vaccination should not be given to
    • Immunocompromised persons, except HIV-infected individuals (see General Principles above)
    • Pregnant women
    • Patients with egg allergy

    3. Rubella
        a. General considerations
            i. Efficacy of vaccine is at least 95%
            ii. Immunization should be given to adults without
                proof of inoculation on or after first birthday or
                without serologic evidence of immunity
        b. Primary series is a single inoculation
        c. Booster dose is not necessary, but it is given coinciden-
           tally with second inoculation for measles
        d. Special considerations
            i. Vaccination should not be given to
                (a) Immunocompromised persons, except HIV-
                    infected individuals (see General Principles
                    above)
                (b) Pregnant women
                (c) Women wishing to become pregnant within 3
                    months of vaccination
                (d) Patients with egg allergy
 C. **Poliomyelitis**
    1. General considerations
        a. Efficacy is at least 95% for either vaccine
        b. Two types of vaccines are available
            i. Enhanced-potency inactivated polio virus (eIPV) is
               preferred for primary series in adults
            ii. Oral live poliovirus vaccine (OPV) is preferred if
                protection within <4 wk is necessary, followed by
                completing primary series as stated below
    2. Primary series
        a. eIPV is given in 3 doses with doses 1 and 2 given 4–8 wk
           apart and dose 3 given within 6–12 mo of dose 2
        b. OPV is given in 3 doses with doses 1 and 2 given 6–8 wk
           apart and dose 3 given within 6 wk–12 mo of dose 2
    3. Booster dose of either eIPV or OPV should be given once
       only to persons who travel in developing countries
    4. Special considerations
        a. OPV, a live virus, should not be given to
            i. Pregnant women
            ii. Those who are immunosuppressed, including pa-
                tients with HIV infection
 D. **Pneumococcal polysaccharide**
    1. General considerations
        a. Covers 23 types of *S. pneumoniae*
            i. Efficacy is estimated at about 60–80% but may be
               lower in some groups (e.g., elderly or those with
               depressed immunity)
        b. Indications for immunization
            i. Age 65 or older
            ii. Persons with the following conditions
                • Chronic liver or renal disease

- Nephrotic syndrome
- Cardiovascular disease
- Chronic respiratory disease
- Diabetes mellitus
- Asplenia
- Alcoholism
- Leukemia, lymphomas or myeloma
- HIV infection and AIDS
- Chronic CSF leak

    iii. Persons living in institutions
    iv. Persons receiving long-term immunosuppressive therapy

  2. Primary series is a single inoculation
  3. Booster dose may be given once to high-risk patients 6 or more years after first dose

E. Hepatitis B
  1. Indications for immunization
    a. Male homosexuals or bisexuals
    b. Intravenous drug users
    c. Intimate family contacts of hepatitis B carriers and intravenous drug users
    d. Mentally impaired persons in institutions
    e. Sexually promiscuous persons
    f. Persons receiving dialysis
    g. Hemophiliacs
    h. Healthcare workers, including those who work with institutionalized mentally impaired persons
    i. Morticians
    j. Persons who travel for >6 mo in endemic areas of the world
    k. Within 7 days after percutaneous or mucous-membrane exposure to HBsAg-infected blood products or within 14 d of sexual exposure to HBsAg-infected person (in either case, vaccine is given with hepatitis B Ig)
  2. Primary series is 3 inoculations, with doses 1 and 2 given 4 wk apart and dose 3 given 5 mo after dose 2
  3. Booster dose may be given 7 yr or more following primary series

F. **Influenza**
  1. See chapter on "Influenza" for details of immuno- and chemoprophylaxis

G. **Immunoglobulins**
  1. Hepatitis A prophylaxis
    a. For travelers to endemic areas, a single IM dose of
      i. 0.02 ml/kg for 2–3 mo of prophylaxis
      ii. 0.06 ml/kg for 5 mo of prophylaxis
    b. For prophylaxis after known exposure to hepatitis A, give a single IM dose of 0.02 ml/kg within 2 wk of exposure

    2. Measles prophylaxis
       a. For non-immune persons
          i. 0.25 ml/kg (maximum of 15 ml) given within 6 d after contact with measles
          ii. Persons who receive measles prophylaxis should get MMR inoculation 3 mo after immunoglobulin
    3. Hepatitis B immune globulin (HBIG)
       a. For non-immune persons exposed to hepatitis B through infected blood or by sexual contact
          i. 5 ml, IM, at different site from primary HB vaccination
          ii. Repeat doses should be given if HB primary series has not yet begun at 1 mo for persons who have had percutaneous or mucous-membrane exposures or at 3 mo for persons who have had sexual exposure

H. Tetanus immune globulin (TIG)
    1. Single dose of 250 U IM is given for unclean, nonminor wound if a patient
       a. Has an unknown tetanus vaccination history
       b. Had 24 or more hr elapse before being treated for wound
       c. Has a history of only one prior primary vaccination

References

1. Centers for Disease Control: Update on adult immunization: Recommendations of the Immunization Practices Advisory Committee. MMWR 40:(RR-12), 1991.
2. U.S. Preventive Services Task Force: Guide to Clinical Preventive Services. Baltimore, Williams & Wilkins, 1989, pp 215–219, 363–367.

Advice to Travelers

I. General Principles

A. International travelers need information on
    1. How to avoid travelers' diarrhea and what to do if diarrhea occurs
    2. Necessary immunizations
    3. Malaria prophylaxis
    4. How to avoid other infectious diseases, such as STDs and AIDS
    5. Risks of travel with chronic conditions
    6. Problems that may be encountered with high temperatures or excessive sunlight exposure
    7. Problems associated with travel to high altitudes (usually over 8,000–10,000 ft)

B. Recommendations and international requirements for immunizations and malaria prophylaxis are subject to change
   1. For up-to-date recommendations
      a. Call the CDC, by touch-tone phone, at (404) 332-4559
      b. Also available are
         i. *Health Information for International Travel,* updated annually, from
            • Centers for Disease Control
              Superintendents of Documents
              US Government Printing Office
              Washington, DC 20402
         ii. *Summary of Health Information for International Travel,* which has biweekly updates, from
            • Division of Quarantine
              Centers for Disease Control
              Atlanta, GA 30333
C. Some health insurance policies may not cover medical expenses and/or transportation back to the U.S. if illness or injury occurs in a foreign country
   1. Advise travelers to ensure that they are covered in the event of medical need or emergency

II. Diagnostics and Evaluation

A. Traveler's itinerary
B. Duration of stay
C. Medical history
D. History of previous immunizations
E. Risk factors associated with travel-related illness
   1. Visiting for more than 4 weeks in areas with poor sanitation
   2. Age (20–29)
   3. Lifestyle while abroad
      a. Living with indigenous populations
      b. Sleeping in tents or boarding houses
   4. History of smoking, chronic gastrointestinal, pulmonary or endocrine illness
   5. Travel to West Africa
   6. Working or studying in the tropics

III. Travelers' Diarrhea

A. General considerations
   1. Episodes are usually self-limited, lasting several days
      a. Most are caused by enterotoxigenic *E. coli*
      b. Persons are also at risk from
         i. *Shigella, Salmonella,* or *Campylobacter* species
         ii. Amoebas
         iii. *Giardia* species
B. Prevention
   1. Restrict diet to cooked foods
   2. Avoid dairy products and peeled fruits and vegetables

3. Avoid food from street vendors
4. Drink only purified or carbonated beverages or drinks made with boiled tap water
5. Avoid ice not made from purified or boiled tap water

C. Prophylaxis
  1. Prophylactic regimens, though not recommended routinely, include any of
    a. Trimethoprim/sulfamethoxazole: 160/800 mg, q.d.
    b. Trimethoprim: 200 mg, q.d.
    c. Doxycycline: 100 mg, one tablet, q.d.
    d. Ciprofloxacin: 500 mg, q.d.
    e. Norfloxacin: 400 mg, q.d.
    f. Pepto-Bismol
      i. Two tablets q.i.d. and q.h.s.
      ii. Can cause mild tinnitus and turns tongue and stool black
      iii. Do not use if traveler is allergic to or is taking salicylates or is taking oral anticoagulants or antibiotics because Pepto-Bismol interferes with absorption

D. Treatment regimens if diarrhea occurs
  1. Hydration with oral replacement salts, purified water, and/or bouillon
  2. Avoid caffeine, ethanol and dairy products
  3. Uncomplicated diarrhea can be controlled with
    a. Loperamide hydrochloride, 4 mg loading dose, then 2 mg after each loose stool, up to a maximum of 16 mg/d
  4. Antibiotic regimen may include one of
    a. Trimethoprim-sulfamethoxazole DS: 800/160 mg b.i.d., for 3 days **or** a single large dose (320/1600 mg)
    b. Ciprofloxacin: 500 mg PO b.i.d. for 3 d
    c. Norfloxacin: 400 mg PO b.i.d. for 3 d

E. Medical attention should be sought if traveler has
  1. Significant dehydration
  2. High fever
  3. Blood in stools
  4. Severe abdominal pain
  5. Persistence of severe diarrhea after treatment

IV. **Immunizations**

A. **General considerations**
  1. More than one vaccine can be given at the same time
    a. Except for cholera and yellow fever vaccines, which should be given at least 3 wk apart
  2. Immunocompromised or pregnant patients should not receive live virus vaccines
    a. HIV-infected persons can and should be immunized against measles, when appropriate

3. Vaccinations to be given should be based on
   a. Risk of exposure in areas of travel
   b. Previous immunization history

B. **Tetanus and diphtheria**
   1. Ensure patient has had primary series and give booster dose if none given in last 10 yr

C. **Poliomyelitis**
   1. Ensure traveler has had primary series
      • See chapter on "Immunizations" for details
   2. For those who have completed a primary series, give booster dose with either live or inactivated polio vaccine

D. **Measles**
   1. Vaccination is recommended for those born after 1956 who have not received two doses of measles vaccine after their first birthday and do not have a physician-documented history of infection or laboratory evidence of immunity
   2. For these individuals, immunize with a single dose of MMR vaccine but do not give at the same time as immune globulin

E. **Hepatitis A**
   1. Advisable for travelers going to areas where hygiene is poor
   2. Immune globulin should be given within 1 month of departure
      a. 2 ml, IM, for a visit of <3 mo
      b. 5 ml, IM, for longer visits
         i. Repeat every 5 mo for continuing coverage

F. **Hepatitis B**
   1. Recommended for travelers who
      a. Are medical personnel whose work could require handling of body fluids
      b. Expect to have sexual contacts, especially in areas that are endemic (Southeast Asia or sub-Saharan Africa)
      c. Expect to travel in areas of high prevalence for 6 or more mo
      d. For details on primary series see previous chapter on "Immunizations"

G. **Cholera**
   1. Vaccine has limited effectiveness and is not often used
      a. Some countries require a single vaccination within 6 mo of entry, if the traveler has visited another country where cholera has been reported

H. **Typhoid**
   1. Efficacy of vaccines is 50–70%
   2. Recommended for travel to rural areas of tropical countries where there are outbreaks or where typhoid is endemic
   3. Two forms of vaccine are available
      a. Live attenuated (oral) vaccine, given at least 2 wk before departure, taking 1 capsule q.o.d. for a total of 4 capsules

      b. Inactivated (injectable) vaccine
          i. Primary series is 2 doses, 0.5 ml each, SQ, given 1 mo apart
          ii. Booster is needed every 3 yr

I. Japanese encephalitis
1. A mosquito-borne disease that occurs in rural Asia
   a. Immunization may be considered for
      i. Summer travelers who spend nights in rural rice-growing areas
      ii. Travelers planning to live in endemic areas
   b. Primary series is 3 doses, SQ, each given 1 wk apart

J. Yellow fever
1. Attenuated live virus vaccine prepared in eggs
2. Recommended for travel to rural areas in the yellow fever endemic zones, including tropical South America and Africa
3. Details from "Summary of Health Information for International Travel" (see above)
4. Vaccine is available only in designated centers
   a. Call local or state health departments for location
5. Boosters are given every 10 yr

K. Meningococcal vaccine
1. Immunization may be advisable for those traveling to Nepal, India, Saudi Arabia, or sub-Saharan Africa

L. Rabies
1. Prophylactic immunization not usually needed prior to travel but should be considered after animal bites
   a. Clean all animal bites thoroughly

V. Malaria Prophylaxis

A. The four Plasmodium species are *Falciparum, Malariae, Vivax,* and *Ovale*
1. Most complications occur from *P. falciparum*

B. Risk of malaria by country is available from the CDC
1. The CDC has information on resistance
2. No drug provides complete protection in all endemic areas
3. Advice from the CDC is available by calling (404) 332-4555
4. Pregnant women should be discouraged from traveling to endemic areas, especially where there is chloroquine-resistant malaria

C. Avoidance of female *Anopheles* mosquitos
1. Wear clothes that cover exposed skin at night
2. Use repellents such as 30% diethyl-metatoluamide (DEET)
3. Sleep under netting or in screened areas

D. Chemoprophylaxis
1. For travel to areas where there is chloroquine-sensitive *P. falciparum*
   a. Chloroquine (base) 300 mg, take once a wk beginning 2 wk prior to travel and continue for 6 wk after exposure risk has ended

2. For travel to areas with chloroquine-resistant species
   a. Mefloquine is preferred prophylactic drug
   b. Alternatively traveler can take chloroquine (as above) and Fansidar (3 tablets to be taken if febrile illness develops and medical care is not immediately available)
3. For specific advice for malaria areas, call the CDC for details

VI. Travel by Persons with Chronic Illnesses

A. General considerations
   1. List generic name of drugs in the event that medications are lost
   2. Needed medications should not be sent in luggage because of the potential for theft or lost or delayed luggage
   3. Carry enough medication to last the entire trip
   4. Patients with cardiovascular or respiratory disease should discuss with physicians any relevant risks associated with travel and/or exertion at higher altitudes

VII. High Altitude Sickness

A. Usually caused by rapidly ascending to altitudes higher than 9,000–12,000 ft
B. Acclimatization for several days at lower altitudes should be considered
C. Common symptoms include nausea, vomiting, fatigue and headache
D. Pulmonary or cerebral edema may be lethal complications of acute mountain sickness
E. For persons who wish to rapidly ascend to high altitudes, consider use of acetazolamide 250 mg b.i.d.–t.i.d., beginning 1–2 d prior to ascent and continuing for several days during ascent
F. Altitude sickness should be treated by descent to lower altitudes and by medical attention if traveler is seriously ill

VIII. Sexually Transmitted Diseases and HIV Infection

A. Travelers should be warned that STDs flourish in all areas of the world
B. Heterosexual transmission of HIV is common in many countries
   1. Very high infection rates are common among prostitutes
   2. Abstinence should be advised
      a. Men at risk should use condoms, preferably those made in countries where quality control is high
      b. Women at risk should use a barrier method of contraception with spermicide and insist that partners use a condom
C. In many developing countries HIV infection may occur from
   1. Injections with nonsterile needles
   2. Blood transfusions

References

1. Advice for travelers. Med Lett 34:41–44, 1992.
2. Frenchick G, Havliche D: Primary prevention and international travel: Infections, immunizations, and antimicrobial prophylaxis. J Gen Intern Med 4:247–258, 1989.
3. Hill D, Pearson R: Health advice for international travel. Ann Intern Med 108:839–852, 1988.

PART V
PRESURGICAL EVALUATION

Outpatient Evaluation of the Surgical Patient: Medical Consultation

I. **General Principles**

   A. The **complete** medical consult may include
1. A complete and directed history and physical, including mental status in geriatric patients
2. Diagnostic tests as indicated by clinical evaluation
3. Identification of patient factors that could increase risk
4. An assessment of the risk-benefit ratio of an operation
   a. Quantify risk by percent of mortality or morbidity whenever possible
   b. This is usually done with the surgeon and/or anesthesiologist
5. Clear recommendations on how to minimize the surgical risk

   B. **Risk categories for mortality**
1. 0–0.01%:   low (usual) risk of mortality
2. 0.01–0.9%:   low but increased risk
3. 1.0–5%:   significant risk
4. 5.0–10%:   moderate risk
5. 10.0–20.0%: high risk of mortality
6. >20%:   very high risk
7. For emergency procedures, double the above percentages for approximate risk of mortality

   C. **Perioperative deaths occur in approximately 0.3% of all operations** with the percentages as follows
1. 10% of deaths occur during induction of anesthesia
   a. Hypoxia is the cause in half of these
2. 35% occur intraoperatively
3. 55% occur within 48 hr postoperatively
   a. Causes include
      i. Inadequate ventilation
      ii. Aspiration
      iii. Arrhythmias
      iv. Drug-related myocardial suppression
      v. Hypotension

   D. **Postoperative deaths** after initial postsurgical period are predominantly caused by

1. Nonpulmonary infections (peritonitis, gram-negative sepsis)
2. Cardiac arrest
3. Pulmonary embolism
4. Renal failure
5. Hypovolemic shock
6. Cancer-related disease
7. Cerebrovascular accident

E. **Preoperative risk** may be divided into 4 categories
   1. **Patient-related** is often subdivided into organ systems
   2. **Procedure-related**
      a. High risk
         i. Craniotomy
         ii. Heart surgery
         iii. Exploratory laparotomy
         iv. Large bowel surgery
      b. Low risk
         i. Cystoscopy
         ii. Hernia repair
         iii. Eye surgery
         iv. D&C, hysterectomy
         v. Plastic surgery
         vi. Oral surgery
   3. **Provider-related**
      a. Depends on experience of surgical team
      b. Consult mortality and morbidity ratios for surgeon(s) and hospital
   4. **Anesthetic-related**
      a. Anesthetic agents are rarely fatal
      b. Most deaths are due to human error
      c. Spinal and general anesthesia have similar degrees of risk associated with their use

II. **Diagnostics**

A. History and physical examination are tailored to the surgical procedure
   • For specific categories refer to subchapters
B. Laboratory data
   1. No definitive consensus is available on routine data for the low- or average-risk surgical patient
   2. Some practitioners will routinely include any of
      a. Electrocardiogram
      b. CBC and differential
      c. Electrolytes, creatinine and BUN
      d. Prothrombin and partial thromboplastin time
      e. Urinalysis
      f. CXR
   3. Most practitioners base necessary laboratory data on
      a. Medical history of the patient
      b. Past laboratory data on the patient

    c. Specifics of the surgical procedure
    d. Requests from the surgeon or surgical center

III. **Management**
  A. **Consultations should address the following**
    1. Diagnosis and problem list
    2. Prognosis and anesthetic and surgical risk are listed by body systems
    3. Does the overall risk outweigh benefits of surgery
    4. Management regimen that decreases the risks
    5. Review of medications
      a. Recommendations on those that will need discontinuation in perioperative period
        • See chapter on "Medications" for details
    6. Whether prophylactic antibiotics are required and, if so, which one(s)
    7. Whether DVT prophylaxis is required and if so, what type
  B. **Suggestions for enhancing implementation**
    1. Address the specific question(s) asked
    2. Limit advice to at most 5 recommendations
    3. Focus on crucial recommendations
    4. Be as specific and exact as possible
      a. Drug dosage, route of administration
      b. Frequency of dose or intervention
    5. Avoid recommending complicated diagnostics or labor intensive procedures if they are not absolutely necessary (if so, do them yourself, after obtaining permission)
    6. Communicate suggestions in person or by phone
    7. Follow-up visits enhance implementation of suggestions and further ensure pre- and postoperative care

Reference

Kroenke MK: Preoperative evaluation: The assessment and management of surgical risk. J Gen Intern Med 2:257–269, 1987.

Preoperative Assessment: Cardiac Risks of Noncardiac Surgery

I. **General Principles**
  A. Most preoperative evaluations done by internists involve risk assessment of only noncardiac surgery because patients undergoing cardiac surgery are almost exclusively evaluated by cardiologists and surgeons

B. **No consensus is available** regarding the preoperative assessment of cardiac risks of noncardiac surgery, and the following is an overview based on reviews

C. **Risk of coronary artery disease**
   1. Many postoperative MIs are silent events with peak occurrence at 3–5 d postoperatively
   2. History of rheumatic fever is not associated with significantly increased risk
   3. History of chronic stable angina and absence of previous MI is not necessarily associated with increased surgical risk but antianginals must be continued throughout perioperative course
   4. Unstable angina indicates very high risk
   5. For persons with a history of MI, but not within past 6 mo, surgical risk increases 5% over baseline rate
   6. Prior CABG is not in itself associated with an increased surgical risk

D. **Risk in congestive heart failure** (CHF)
   1. Decompensated CHF (JVD or S3) is associated with increased risk
   2. History of pulmonary edema within 1 wk of surgery is associated with a significantly increased risk
   3. Compensated CHF (without evidence of S3 or a raised JVP) is associated with a small increased risk, but much less than decompensated CHF

E. Risks of other cardiac- and cardiovascular-related problems
   1. **Peripheral, aortic, or carotid vascular disease** is highly associated with cardiac morbidity and mortality
   2. **Arrhythmias**
      a. Supraventricular tachycardias (SVTs) are common, regardless of the presence or absence of CAD
      b. >5 PVCs or PACs per min may be associated with increased risk
      c. Heart disease of any cause increases the risk of life-threatening arrhythmias
   3. Hypertension is not a surgical risk factor if hypertension is controlled and there is no end organ damage

F. **The Goldman criteria** (listed in order of decreasing significance) are frequently used to quantify cardiac risk (Table 1)

G. **The Eagle criteria** may also assist in determination of risk for peripheral vascular surgical procedures
   1. Risk factors
      a. Age >70
      b. Diabetes mellitus
      c. Angina
      d. Q waves on EKG
      e. Ventricular arrhythmias
   2. A score of 1 or 2 risk factors is considered intermediate risk, while 3 or more is considered high risk

TABLE 1. The Goldman Criteria

Factors		Points
1	S3 gallop or elevated JVD	11
2	MI within last 6 mo	10
3	Rhythm other than sinus or sinus plus presence of PACs on last preoperative EKG	7
4	Presence >5 PVCs/min	7
5	Age >70	5
6	Emergency surgery	4
7	Significant aortic stenosis (by examination or echocardiogram)	3
8	Intraperitoneal, intrathoracic or aortic operation	3
9	Any one of: PO_2 <60, PCO_2 >50 mmHg, K <3.0, HCO_3 <20, BUN >50, Cr >3.0, abnormal SGOT or chronic liver disease, patient bedridden due to noncardiac cause (Maximum is 3 points regardless of number of abnormalities found above)	3
	Total points	53

Goldman Classes	Risk of Major Complications (%)*	Risk of Cardiac Death (%)
I = 0–5 pts	0.7	0.2
II = 6–12 pts	5.0	2.0
III = 13–25 pts	12.0	2.0
IV = 26 pts or greater	22.0	56.0

* Major complications refer to intraoperative or postoperative MI, pulmonary edema, or nonfatal ventricular tachycardia

II. **Diagnostics**

  A. **History**
   1. Presence or absence of Goldman criteria listed above
   2. Anginal symptoms or equivalent
   3. Symptoms of CHF (orthopnea, paroxysmal nocturnal dyspnea, shortness of breath, swelling of ankles)
   4. Exercise tolerance (i.e., walking distance, stair climbing)
   5. Other vascular symptoms, including intermittent claudication and transient ischemic attacks
   6. Smoking history and alcohol use
   7. Medications for control of angina, hypertension, and/or arrhythmias
   8. Previous surgical history and complications, if any
  B. **Examination**
   1. General physical and mental status
   2. Cardiac and respiratory examinations for indications of heart failure
   3. Presence of carotid or abdominal bruits
   4. Extremity examination for changes of peripheral vascular disease
  C. **Laboratory data**
   1. For those at risk of cardiac complications

          a. Electrocardiogram
          b. Electrolytes, creatinine, and BUN
          c. Liver function tests for use in Goldman criteria
          d. Urinalysis
      2. Additional data for selected patients
          a. Complete blood count for anemia
          b. Metabolites: calcium, phosphorus, magnesium
          c. Arterial blood gas
          d. Dipyridamole–thallium study should be considered for patients with 1 or more risk factors as determined by Eagle criteria
          e. Radionuclide ventriculography (MUGA) may be considered for quantification of ejection fraction in persons with congestive heart failure
             i. Ejection fraction does not, however, predict postoperative cardiac risks
          f. Echocardiography should be considered for assessment of suspected valvular disease and ventricular function or evaluation of gradient across involved valve(s) when valvular disease is potentially significant

   D. **Further evaluations for specific surgery**
      1. Noncardiac vascular surgery
          a. A Goldman score >12 or an Eagle score ≥ 3 (for vascular surgery) confers a higher risk of postoperative myocardial infarction and cardiac death
          b. Selected patients should be considered for preoperative noninvasive cardiac testing by one or more of
             i. Exercise tolerance testing
            ii. Dipyridamole–thallium scintigraphy
          c. For positive test results on either investigation, consider myocardial revascularization prior to surgery, especially if results indicate ischemia in 3 coronary artery areas
          d. Refer to cardiology for consideration of angiography and further evaluation

III. **Management**

   A. **General approach**
      1. Patients at high risk for postoperative cardiac complications as determined by Goldman and/or Eagle criteria should be strongly considered for invasive cardiac monitoring
      2. Patients who should be considered for coronary revascularization prior to other vascular surgery
          a. Those whose ischemic pattern indicates that revascularization or PTCA will increase life expectancy
          b. Those who have angina that is difficult to control with medication

   B. **For hypertensive patients**
      1. If diastolic blood pressure >110 mmHg

      a. Evaluate for end-organ damage

      b. Establish control of blood pressure before recommending elective surgery

  2. Continue antihypertensives except for diuretics on day of operation

  3. If the patient is NPO for more than 12–24 hr, consider recommending parenteral antihypertensives until patient is able to tolerate oral medications

C. **For recent myocardial infarct**

  1. Avoid elective surgery within 6 mo of an MI

  2. Urgent surgeries can be done sooner, but patient may need invasive monitoring

  3. If electrocardiographic data are consistent with an MI of unknown duration (i.e., a silent MI), avoid elective surgery for 6 mo and consider a cardiac evaluation with

      a. Exercise tolerance test or dipyridamole–thallium study

      b. Echocardiography to detect segmental ventricular wall motion abnormalities

D. **For congestive heart failure**

  1. Patients should be managed to resolve or minimize CHF prior to surgery

  2. Patients with low ejection fractions may need invasive monitoring perioperatively

  3. Medications for CHF should be continued throughout the postoperative period

E. **For valvular heart disease**

  1. Rate control and maintenance of normal sinus rhythm, if possible, are of utmost importance in mitral stenosis

  2. Endocarditis prophylaxis may be appropriate

     • Refer to chapter on "Endocarditis"

  3. Patients with significant valvular disease should have echocardiography

      a. Consult cardiology for further management and/or monitoring perioperatively

F. **For patients on anticoagulation therapy** consider either of 2 strategies

  1. Discontinue oral anticoagulant 3 d before surgery and cover patient with heparin prior to and after surgery; this is especially important in patients who are at high risk when not anticoagulated; for instance, those with

      a. Prosthetic mitral valves

      b. Recent or recurrent thromboembolic episode

      c. Hypercoagulable states (e.g., lupus anticoagulant)

  2. Discontinue oral anticoagulants 1–3 d preoperatively; surgery may commence when PT is normal or 1 sec above control; oral anticoagulants are resumed 1–3 d postoperatively

G. **For patients with pacemakers**

  1. These patients should have referral to cardiology for evaluation of pacemaker and battery pre- and postoperatively

IV. **Referrals to Cardiology Prior to Surgery for**

    A. Uncertainty of presurgical risk assessment

    B. Evaluation for myocardial revascularization

    C. Evaluation of significant valvular disease as indicated by clinical evaluation or echocardiogram

    D. Assessment of pacemaker function

    E. Unstable angina or angina-equivalent

    F. For high-risk patients who need invasive monitoring prior to and/or following surgery

References

1. Eagle KA, Coley CM, Newell JB, et al: Combining clinical and thallium data optimizes preoperative assessment of cardiac risk before vascular surgery. Ann Intern Med 110:859–866, 1989.
2. Goldman L: Cardiac risks and complications of noncardiac surgery. Ann Intern Med 98:504–513, 1983.
3. Granieri R, Macpherson DS: Preoperative care of the vascular surgery patient: The perspective of the internist. J Gen Intern Med 7:102–113, 1992.
4. Kroenke MK: Preoperative evaluation: The assessment and management of surgical risk. J Gen Intern Med 2:257–269, 1987.
5. Wong T, Detsky AS: Preoperative cardiac risk assessment for patients having peripheral vascular surgery. Ann Intern Med 116:743–753, 1992.

Deep Vein Thrombosis Prophylaxis

I. **General Principles**

    A. Prophylaxis needs to be considered for the following persons undergoing major surgical procedures

       1. All patients >40 y/o

       2. Patients <40 y/o with one or more of the following risk factors for thrombosis

          a. Hypercoagulable state (e.g., malignancy, lupus anticoagulant)

          b. Stasis

             i. Heart failure

             ii. Myocardial infarction

             iii. Anasarca

          c. Obesity

          d. Immobilization

          e. Estrogen therapy

          f. Sepsis

          g. Prior thromboembolic events

    B. Postoperative DVTs occur in up to 25% of persons undergoing general, urologic, gynecologic, neurologic, and orthopedic surgery

    C. Postoperative DVTs may occur in up to 40% of those under-going hip surgery, knee reconstruction, gynecologic cancer operations, open prostatectomies, major neurosurgical procedures

    D. Mortality from pulmonary embolism ranges from 1–5% depending on patient characteristics and surgical procedure

II. **Diagnostics**

    A. **History and physical examination** should evaluate presence of above factors for patients undergoing major surgery

    B. **Laboratory data**
        1. For patients on or being considered for anticoagulation
           a. Prothrombin time and/or partial thromboplastin time

III. **Management**

    A. The consulting physician should:
        1. Evaluate potential risk for DVT in a particular patient
        2. Ascertain risk of DVT for the surgical procedure
        3. Discuss with patient the risks of DVT

    B. **Prophylaxis** is usually continued until
        1. 5–7 d postoperatively or when patient is mobile and/or discharged from hospital

    C. **General recommendations**
        1. Cessation of smoking prior to surgery
        2. Cessation of estrogen prior to surgery
           a. This should be discussed with the surgeon
        3. Weight reduction in overweight patients before elective surgery

    D. **Common methods of prophylaxis**
        1. **Oral anticoagulation**
           a. Two-step Coumadin
               i. Begin 10 d before surgery
               ii. Keep PT 2–3 sec above initial baseline
               iii. Dose is adjusted after surgery to increase PT 1.5 times the control level
           b. Low-dose Coumadin
               i. Patient started on low-dose Coumadin with PT kept at 2–3 sec above baseline
        2. **Heparinization methods** used in hospital
           a. Low-dose heparin is 5000 U SQ, b.i.d. to t.i.d.
           b. Adjusted-dose heparin is begun 2 days before surgery at 3,500 U SQ t.i.d. with PTT kept in 30–40 sec range
        3. **Pneumatic compression**
           a. Intermittent pressure is applied to lower limbs by means of inflatable leggings
        4. **Dextran infusion**
           a. Used prior to and during surgery, but must be used cautiously in patients prone to CHF
           b. Side effects include skin rashes, anaphylaxis, and decreased renal function

F. **General methods of prophylaxis for specific surgical procedures**
  1. **General abdominal surgery**
     a. Low-dose heparin
     b. Pneumatic compression
  2. **Urologic surgery**
     a. Low-dose heparin except for open prostatectomies, in which adjusted-dose heparin is recommended
     b. External pneumatic compression
  3. **Gynecologic surgery**
     a. Low-dose heparin is usually used except for gynecologic cancers, for which adjusted-dose heparin is recommended
  4. **Orthopedic (hips and knees) surgery**
     a. Any of the following may be used
        i. Adjusted-dose heparin
        ii. Two-step warfarin
        iii. One-step warfarin
        iv. External pneumatic compression
        v. Dextran
  5. **Neurosurgery, head and neck surgery**
     a. Intracranial surgery: external pneumatic compression
     b. Extracranial surgery: low-dose heparin
  6. **Lower extremity surgery**
     a. Low-dose heparin

Reference

Kroenke MK: Preoperative evaluation: The assessment and management of surgical risk. J Gen Intern Med 2:257–269, 1987.

Diabetes Mellitus in the Perioperative Period

I. **General Principles**
  A. **Diabetics** more commonly have comorbidities such as
     1. Cardiac and peripheral vascular disease
     2. Renal insufficiency
     3. Obesity
  B. **Atherosclerotic vascular disease and infection** cause the vast majority of morbidity and mortality
  C. Patients with evidence of **autonomic neuropathy** that affects heart rate are at increased risk for perioperative cardiac morbidity and mortality
  D. **Hypoglycemia** is more likely to occur intraoperatively or around 4–6 d postoperatively when insulin requirements start to decrease

E. **Goals of perioperative care**
   1. Control of blood glucose prior to elective surgery should consistently be <180 mg/dl
   2. Evaluate comorbidities
   3. Reduce risk from diabetes and comorbidities
   4. Inform surgeon of relevant laboratory data and medical risks of surgery

II. **Diagnostics**

A. **History**
   1. Age of onset of diabetes
   2. Medications
   3. Methods and frequency of monitoring blood glucose
   4. History of treatment for ketoacidosis or hyperosmolar condition
   5. Hyperglycemic symptoms
      a. Polyuria, polydipsia, and/or polyphagia
      b. Weight loss
      c. Postural lightheadedness
   6. Complications from diabetic disorder
      a. Paresthesias and sensory loss in lower extremities
      b. Leg or foot ulcers
      c. Occult infections
      d. Visual symptoms
   7. Presence of comorbid symptoms/disease
      a. Vascular diseases
         i. Angina or anginal equivalent
         ii. TIAs
         iii. Intermittent claudication
      b. Congestive heart failure

B. **Examination**
   1. General for volume status (mucous membranes, skin tenting, orthostasis)
   2. Cardiovascular examination includes assessment for autonomic neuropathy
      a. Orthostatic measurements (BP and pulse), supine, and standing, at 30 sec and 3–5 min
      b. Heart response to mild exercise if patient initially has pulse rate <50 beats/min at rest (abnormal variation is increase of <5 beats/min between maximum and minimum pulse)
      c. Signs of peripheral vascular disease
      d. Carotid and abdominal bruits
   3. Neurological examination
      a. Peripheral neuropathy
      b. Signs of old CVA
   4. Extremities examination
      a. Leg and foot ulcers

C. **Laboratory data**
1. Initial investigations
   a. Serum glucose (fasting)
   b. Glycosylated hemoglobin
   c. Complete blood count
   d. Electrolytes and anion gap calculation
   e. Creatinine and BUN
   f. Electrocardiogram
      i. Look for evidence of old MI/silent MI
   g. Urinalysis

III. **Management**

A. **General approach**
1. Blood glucose and electrolytes should be monitored closely perioperatively to avoid complications such as DKA and poor wound healing
2. Blood glucose control is important to maximize WBC function and minimize volume depletion from polyuria
3. If patient needs contrast radiography, then ensure that patient is well hydrated prior to procedure
4. If patient has symptoms of vascular disease(s), he/she may need evaluation and investigation prior to other elective surgical procedures
   • See chapter on "Cardiac Risks of Noncardiac Surgery"

B. **For selected situations**
1. **If patient is on oral hypoglycemic therapy**
   a. Chlorpropamide should be discontinued 3 d prior to surgery
   b. Glipizide and glyburide should be discontinued the night before surgery
   c. Monitor blood glucose perioperatively by chemstrips and reduce high blood glucose with regular insulin
   d. Restart medications once patient is on usual diet
   e. Alternatives for minor day surgery
      i. Holding oral hypoglycemic on day of surgery
      ii. Dextrose infusion and monitoring perioperatively
      iii. Restarting oral hypoglycemic next morning when patient on usual diet
   f. **For major surgery**
      i. Patient will likely need sliding scale with regular insulin every 6 hr, keeping blood glucose below 180 mg/dl
2. **For diabetics requiring insulin**
   a. **General approach**
      i. Attempt to schedule surgery early in the day
      ii. Admit patient prior to surgery and monitor perioperatively
   b. **For minor day surgery, consider**
      i. Scheduling surgery early in the day

        ii. Giving $1/3$ to $1/2$ of usual morning dose of NPH insulin and holding regular insulin

       iii. Checking morning blood glucose

       iv. Giving dextrose IV preoperatively

       v. Monitoring blood glucose postoperatively

      vi. Having patient resume normal diet with modified insulin coverage on day of surgery

      vii. Resuming usual insulin dosing when patient is on usual diet

  c. **For major surgery**

    i. Admit prior to procedure

IV. **Referral to Endocrinologist for**

  A. Uncertainty of management

  B. Difficulty in controlling fragile diabetic

References

1. Cygan R, Waitzkin H: Stopping and restarting medications in the perioperative period. J Gen Intern Med 2:270–283, 1987.
2. Kroenke K: The assessment of surgical risk. J Gen Intern Med 2:257–269, 1987.

Medications in the Perioperative Period

I. **General Principles**

  A. Medications in use by the patient may present problems during or after a major surgical procedure

  B. Most medications may be continued if surgery is minor and/or done on a day surgery or overnight basis

  C. Discuss with surgeon and/or anesthesiologist and/or pharmacist for details

  D. Some medications may need modification or substitution depending on

    1. Type of drug

    2. Surgical procedure

    3. Patient's ability to take oral medications

II. **Psychiatric Medications**

  A. **Antidepressants**

    1. Tricyclic antidepressants may interfere with anesthesia by potentiating CNS depression

    2. Monoamine oxidase inhibitors may cause hypertensive crises

    3. Recommendations for most patients

      a. Stop either type of antidepressant several days to one week prior to surgery

      b. Restart after patient is stable postoperatively

B. **Antipsychotics**
   1. May cause hypotension and myocardial depression, especially thorazine
   2. Recommendations for most patients
      a. Stop several days prior to surgery
      b. Restart once patient is stable postoperatively
C. **Lithium**
   1. Recommendations for most patients is to taper (usually over 1 wk) and discontinue several days prior to surgery
D. **Tranquilizers**
   1. Whenever possible, discontinue several days prior to surgery to avoid increasing anesthetic risks

III. **Nonsteroidal Anti-inflammatory Drugs (NSAIDs)**

   A. **Aspirin and aspirin-containing medications**
      1. May prolong bleeding time
      2. Recommendation is to discontinue at least 1 wk before surgery
   B. **Other NSAIDs**
      1. Cause reversible antiplatelet effects
      2. May cause worsening of renal function if taken chronically
      3. Recommendation is to stop NSAID prior to surgery
         a. Time of discontinuation depends on half-life of specific drug; e.g.
            i. Piroxicam (Feldene) should be stopped 1 wk prior to surgery
            ii. Ibuprofen may be stopped the day prior to surgery

IV. **Medication for Endocrine Disorders**

   A. **Insulin:** recommendations
      1. ½ dose of usual NPH (or equivalent) on morning of surgery
      2. Dextrose infusion used perioperatively
      3. Sliding scale with regular insulin until patient is stable and is taking usual diet
   B. **Oral hypoglycemics**
      1. Recommendations for most patients
         a. For long-acting oral hypoglycemics such as chlorpropamide, stop 3 d preoperatively
         b. For short-acting oral hypoglycemics such as glyburide and glipizide, stop day before surgery
      2. Blood glucose measurements
         a. Measure blood glucose on morning of surgery
         b. Monitor every 6 hr until patient on usual diet
      3. Alternatively for day surgery, consider
         a. Use of dextrose infusion for duration of surgery
         b. Monitor periodically until patient discharged
         c. Advise patient to take usual diet
         d. Restart oral hypoglycemic the following morning if patient on usual diet

C. **Corticosteroids**
   1. **Adrenal suppression occurs with**
      a. Chronic use at dose above prednisone 7.5 mg q.d. (or other corticosteroid equivalent)
      b. High-dose daily steroids for >7 d
      c. High-dose alternate-day steroids
   2. **Adrenal suppression may occur with**
      a. Short courses of high-dose steroids
      b. Chronic low-dose steroids
   3. **Recommendations for most persons**
      a. If there is any question of adrenal suppression, consider ACTH stimulation test prior to surgery
      b. If adrenal suppression is likely or an ACTH stimulation test is unavailable before surgery for a patient who may have adrenal suppression, patient will need hydrocortisone IV in perioperative period
         i. Dose: 100 mg IV q 8 or equivalent corticosteroid
D. **Thyroid medications**
   1. Levothyroxine
      a. Levothyroxine is long acting and can be withheld, if necessary, for up to 1 wk before adverse effects occur
      b. Recommendations for elective surgery in hypothyroid patients
         i. If patient is not clinically euthyroid, reschedule elective surgery and correct with thyroid replacement therapy
         ii. If patient is clinically euthyroid
            (a) Continue thyroxine until day of surgery
            (b) Restart when able to take oral medications
E. **Estrogens/progestin preparations**
   1. **Oral contraceptive pill (OCP)**
      a. May increase the risk for thromboembolic event
      b. Recommendations for most patients
         i. Consider stopping 3 wk preoperatively
         ii. Restart OCP with next cycle
         iii. Consider DVT prophylaxis with minidose heparin
         iv. Advise patient to use other method of contraception if pregnancy is to be avoided
   2. **Estrogen replacement therapy**
      a. Does not seem to increase the risk for thromboses
      b. Recommendations for most patients is to continue estrogen in perioperative period

V. **Cardiac Medications**

   A. Most cardiac medications should be continued during perioperative period
   B. Do not stop beta blockers
   C. Some practitioners advocate stopping diuretics in order to avoid volume depletion and/or hypokalemia

VI. Anticoagulation

A. General approach
1. Choice of whether to discontinue anticoagulation depends on
   a. Danger to patient if anticoagulation is stopped
   b. Potential for bleeding and complications from bleeding for a given surgical procedure
2. Decision to stop anticoagulation entirely or substitute heparin in the perioperative period should be undertaken in consultation with surgeon and patient

B. Stopping anticoagulation entirely in the perioperative period may be hazardous for patients with a history of
1. Prosthetic heart valve
2. Recurrent or recent thromboembolic event(s)
3. Hypercoagulable states (e.g., lupus anticoagulant)

C. Two alternative approaches for elective surgery
1. Discontinue oral anticoagulation several days prior to surgery
   a. Restart oral anticoagulation 1–3 d postoperatively
2. Cover patient with IV heparin until prothrombin time can be restabilized postoperatively

VII. Antiepileptics

A. Continue therapy and check drug level(s) preoperatively

Reference

Cygan R, Waitzkin H: Stopping and restarting medications in the perioperative period. J Gen Intern Med 2:270–283, 1987.

Surgical Risks in Obese Patients

I. Definition

A. Obesity is defined as $>30\%$ over desirable body weight

II. General Principles

A. The obese patient is considered more susceptible to postoperative complications, although few prospective studies of the extent of the risk have been done
B. There is little documented evidence to justify denying surgery in the obese patient based on weight alone, and the usual risk and benefits need to be analyzed

III. Surgical Risk

A. **Anesthesia**

1. Chief concerns include
   a. Venous access
   b. Maintaining adequate ventilation
2. Obese patients do not have an increased morbidity due to anesthetic agents

B. **Pulmonary**
  1. Smoking compounds risk with obese patients
  2. Obese patients with >30% of predicted weight may have a significant decrease in
     a. Vital capacity and residual volume
     b. Expiratory reserve
     c. Total lung capacity
     d. Maximum voluntary ventilation
  3. Atelectasis, ventilation, and perfusion mismatching are common, especially in the older obese patient
  4. Hypoventilation syndrome occurs in <10% of obese patients

C. **Cardiovascular**
  1. Obesity predisposes to cardiovascular morbidity (as noted in the Framingham study)
  2. The morbidly obese patient often has
     a. Significant deterioration of cardiac function intraoperatively
     b. Delayed cardiac recuperation

D. **Thromboembolic disease**
  1. Pulmonary embolism is a more frequent cause of postoperative deaths in the obese patient than in the nonobese patient
  2. Thrombophlebitis is also more common in the obese

E. **Wound healing**
  1. In general, the obese have an increased risk of wound infections
  2. Excessive subcutaneous fat predisposes to wound seroma, hematomas, infection, wound separation, and hernias

IV. **Diagnostics**

A. **History**
  1. Weight history
  2. Diet
  3. Exercise tolerance
  4. Smoking history
  5. Ability to mobilize
  6. Sleep apnea
  7. Other cardiac and respiratory risks

B. **Examination**
  1. Weight
  2. Site of surgery and amount of gross subcutaneous fat
  3. Skin
     a. Especially around the panniculus and groin area, where Candida is common

b. Varicose veins
4. Lung crackles suggestive of atelectasis
5. Peripheral pulses and sites for venous access

C. **Laboratory data**
   1. For selected patients depending on clinical evaluation and type of surgery
      a. Electrocardiogram
      b. Pulmonary function tests
      c. Arterial blood gas

V. **Management**

A. Prior to elective surgery
   1. Encourage weight loss
      a. Reduction in weight by 10–15% can have dramatic effects on cardiopulmonary and glucose tolerance (if decreased)
      b. Weight loss should not be achieved at the expense of lean body mass (keep protein diet at least 1.5 g/kg of desirable body weight)
   2. Abstain from smoking for a minimum of 4 wk
   3. Teach patient breathing exercises with incentive spirometry

B. Deep venous thrombosis prophylaxis is strongly recommended
   1. See chapter on "DVT Prophylaxis" for details
   2. Encourage early ambulation postoperatively

Reference

Pasulka P, et al: The risks of surgery in obese patients. Ann Intern Med 104:540–546, 1986.

Pulmonary Disease in the Perioperative Period

I. **General Principles**

A. **Chronic obstructive pulmonary disease** (COPD) is an important risk factor for pulmonary complications of surgery because these patients cannot generate an effective cough to clear secretions, leading to a higher incidence of atelectasis and pneumonia

B. **Anesthesia** is associated with factors that further compromise pulmonary function
   1. Decreased functional residual capacity (FRC)
   2. Ventilation-perfusion mismatching
   3. Intrapulmonary shunting
   4. Atelectasis

C. **Other factors that may increase pulmonary risk**
   1. Surgery that impinges on respiratory function

      a. Thoracic surgery

      b. Upper abdominal surgery

    2. Surgical procedures necessitating anesthesia >2–3 hr

    3. Risk increases significantly with persons >70 y/o

    4. Smoking cigarettes

  D. Predictors of increased surgical risk

    1. High risk: FEV_1 <1000 ml

         or

      maximum voluntary ventilation (MVV) <50% of predicted

         or

      $PaCO_2$ >45 mmHg

    2. Medium risk: FEV_1 between 1000 and 2000 ml

    3. Low risk: FEV_1 >2000 ml

II. Diagnostics

  A. History

    1. Smoking history

    2. Environmental/work history

    3. Previous diagnosis of lung disease

      a. COPD with carbon dioxide retention (PCO_2 >45)

      b. Asthma

      c. Restrictive lung disease

      d. Asthmatic and/or chronic bronchitis

    4. History of productive cough or abnormal dyspnea

  B. Examination

    1. Weight

    2. Respiratory evaluation

      a. Respiratory rate

      b. Positive loose cough test

      c. Crackles and/or wheezing

      d. Prolonged expiratory phase

    3. Cardiac examination for right ventricular heave and/or right heart failure

    4. Extremities for

      a. Cyanosis

      b. Edema

  C. Laboratory data

    1. For selected patients with suspicion or evidence of pulmonary disease

      a. Chest x-ray

      b. Complete blood count

      c. Electrolytes

      d. Electrocardiogram

      e. Pulmonary function testing (PFT)

        i. Standard indication for PFT is prior to lung resection

        ii. Further indications for PFTs may include

          (a) Thoracic or upper abdominal surgery in patients with a history of cigarette smoking and/or dyspnea or with known pulmonary disease

            (b) Evaluation of suspected, undiagnosed pulmonary disease

            (c) Evaluation in persons known to retain carbon dioxide

    f. Arterial blood gas analysis should be considered if

        i. Patient has known pulmonary disease

        ii. PFTs indicate pulmonary disease

        iii. Patient has symptoms suggestive of pulmonary disease

        iv. CBC indicates polycythemia

        v. EKG indicates right heart strain

III. Management

A. General approach

    1. Postoperative incentive spirometry should be considered for patients with

      a. Diagnosis or evidence of pulmonary disease

      b. Chronic cough and/or smoking history

      c. Impaired mobility after surgery

      d. Thoracic or upper abdominal surgery

      e. Age >65 and undergoing any major surgical procedure

B. Specific measures may include

    1. Medications continued through perioperative period for patients with bronchospasm

    2. Maximize pulmonary function by

      a. Smoking cessation prior to surgery

      b. Appropriate use of bronchodilators and inhaled or oral steroids

        i. Consider starting steroids prior to admission if patient has had a recent exacerbation

      c. Weight loss for overweight patients

    3. Incentive spirometry and strict pulmonary hygiene are useful postoperatively, with the best results accruing when patient is taught how to use spirometer before surgery

    4. If patient is on steroids, some practitioners increase dose 1 wk preoperatively to stabilize pulmonary status (if necessary)

    5. Patients on steroids or who may have adrenal suppression from previous steroid use need perioperative IV hydrocortisone

      a. Usual dose, 100 mg q 8 hr or equivalent to avoid adrenal crisis

IV. Referrals to a Pulmonary Specialist for

A. Uncertainty of diagnosis or management

B. For severe lung disease

C. Unstable lung disease (e.g., recent exacerbations of asthma or COPD)

D. For patients undergoing lung resection

References

1. American College of Physicians: Preoperative pulmonary function testing. Ann Intern Med 112:793–794, 1990.
2. Jackson CV: Preoperative pulmonary evaluation. Arch Intern Med 148:2120–2127, 1988.
3. Kroenke MK: Preoperative evaluation: The assessment and management of surgical risk. J Gen Intern Med 2:257–269, 1987.
4. Zibrak J, O'Donnell CR, Marton K: Indications of pulmonary function testing. Ann Intern Med 112:763–771, 1990.

PART VI
PRIMARY CARE FOR ADULTS
A

Abdominal Aortic Aneurysms

I. **Definition**

Abdominal aortic aneurysm (AAA) is defined as **infrarenal aorta with transverse diameter** >1.5 × the diameter of the aorta at level of renal arteries (translates to >3 cm in most people)

II. **General Principles**
   A. More common in men than women
   B. Significant cause of death in men >55 y/o
   C. AAAs rarely rupture with girth <5 cm
   D. AAAs grow at estimated rate of 0.2–0.4 cm/yr
   E. General rule
      1. Aneurysms >6 cm need repair
      2. Aneurysms <4 cm can be observed
      3. Aneurysms 4–6 cm = no consensus on intervention
   F. Majority of AAAs are found in asymptomatic individuals
   G. Abdominal palpation has a poor detection rate for AAA (sensitivity <50%)
   H. AAA **must** be in the differential diagnosis of an older person with new onset of back or abdominal pain

III. **Diagnostics**
   A. History
      1. **Positive family history** of AAA in first-degree relative
      2. **Atherosclerotic and other vascular disease:** CAD, PVD
      3. **Sustained hypertension**
      4. **Smoking**
      5. **Symptoms of an expanding AAA**
         a. Abdominal, back, or flank pain
         b. Enlargement of palpable pulsatile abdominal mass
         c. Hematuria, pulsating urination, testicular pain
         d. "Blue-toe" syndrome (from microemboli)
            i. Painful and cyanotic toes on both feet
   B. Examination
      1. **Signs suggestive** of AAA
         a. Nontender pulsatile and/or expansile abdominal mass with or without bruit

        b. Mid or lower abdominal bruit

        c. "Blue-toe" syndrome

    2. Other vascular bruits

    3. Peripheral pulses

   C. **Laboratory data**

     1. **Ultrasound** is used for diagnosis, sizing, and monitoring

        a. The **larger of the transverse or AP diameter** of AAA is used for descriptive and prognostic purposes

        b. **Length** of AAA is **not** generally a consideration in prognosis or for determining intervention

IV. **Management**

   A. **Symptomatic AAA**

     1. Symptomatic or rapidly expanding AAAs are referred urgently

   B. **Asymptomatic AAA**

     1. **General approach**

        a. Evaluation of surgical risks (see below)

        b. Assess size of AAA by ultrasound

        c. Consult or refer to a vascular surgeon

           i. If intervention is warranted, surgeon will request further studies with angiogram and/or CT and MRI

     2. **If surgery is not done** because of size of AAA or patient refusal or if surgical risk is too high

        a. **Repeat ultrasound every 3–6 mo**

        b. **Reconsult** surgeon if

           i. Aneurysm grows rapidly

           ii. Patient develops symptoms (see below)

           iii. Aneurysm becomes larger than a predetermined size (which is often 6 cm), as decided by physician, surgeon, and patient

        c. **Reduce risk factors**

           i. Cease cigarette smoking

           ii. Control hypertension

     3. **Advise patient to seek immediate medical care** in case of

        a. New onset of back pain

        b. Abdominal or flank pain

        c. Enlargement of palpable pulsatile abdominal mass

        d. Hematuria, pulsating urination, testicular pain

        e. Blue-toe syndrome

   C. Special considerations

     1. Assess **renal function** if angiogram is planned

     2. Evaluate potential for **cardiac complications** (see also Goldman criteria, p 35)

        a. For patients with stable, medication-controlled angina, consider presurgical exercise stress test or dipyrimadole–thallium stress test

        b. If stress test is positive for myocardial ischemia, refer for cardiologic evaluation

   D. **Assess carotid circulation** by history and physical
      1. Asymptomatic bruits can be left alone
      2. History of TIAs requires Duplex scan
      3. If stenosis is significant, notify vascular surgeon
        • See chapter on "Carotid Stenosis and Bruits" for details

V. **Referral to Vascular Surgeon**

   A. Urgently if patient has expanding or symptomatic AAA
   B. For initial evaluation, if patient is a surgical candidate
   C. For uncertainty of diagnosis or treatment
   D. For significant, rapid expansion of an asymptomatic AAA

References

1. Editorial: Management of small abdominal aneurysms. Ann Intern Med 113:731, 1990.
2. Reuler JB, Kumar KL: Abdominal aortic aneurysm. J Gen Intern Med 6:360–366, 1991.

Acne

I. **Definition**

Acne vulgaris is a follicular disorder of unknown cause

II. **General Principles**

   A. Prevalence of acne is nearly 10% of U.S. population
   B. Prevalence in adolescents is as high as 85%
   C. Acne often begins in early teens and may extend into adulthood
      1. Frequency is highest in late adolescence
      2. Acne occasionally first appears in persons >30 y/o
   D. Acne is almost always idiopathic but may be secondary to
      1. Medications: anabolic steroids
      2. Disorders: Cushing's syndrome, virilizing conditions
   E. Acne can damage both skin and psyche
   F. Address psychological well-being because what may seem minor to an adult may be extremely distressing to an adolescent

III. **Diagnostics**

   A. **History**
      1. Age at onset
      2. Location (back, face, neck, chest)
      3. Aggravating factors (stress, seasons, cosmetics and creams)
      4. Menstrual history and premenstrual worsening of acne
      5. Previous treatments

      6. Family history of acne

      7. Medications and drug use

B. **Examination**

      1. Location of acne

      2. Type of acneform lesions

          a. Open and/or closed comedones

          b. Papules, pustules, and/or cystic

      3. Severity of disease

      4. Complications (scarring, skin changes)

      5. Evaluation of hirsutism in women

C. **Laboratory data**

      1. Initial investigations: not necessary

      2. Further investigations (if clinical evaluation warrants)

          a. Culture and sensitivity: for folliculitis

          b. Evaluation of hirsutism: see chapter on "Hirsutism"

          c. Skin biopsy: if other skin disease suspected

IV. **Management**

A. For **mild to moderate acne without scarring**

      1. **Topical therapies**

          a. Avoid contact with lips, eyelids, and mucous membranes

          b. Mild astringents and/or cleansers (e.g., pHisoDerm)

          c. Benzoyl peroxide: lotion or gel (2.5%, 5%, 10%), q.h.s.–b.i.d.

          d. Sulfur preparations: Clearasil or Fostex

          e. Antibiotics, q.d.–t.i.d.

             i. Tetracycline: solution

             ii. Clindamycin: solution or gel

             iii. Erythromycin: solution (1.5%, 2%)

             iv. Meclocycline: cream (1%)

          f. **Tretinoin** (Retin A)

             i. Cream (0.05%, 0.1%)

             ii. Gel (0.01%, 0.025%)

             iii. Liquid (0.05%)

             iv. Therapeutic results begin at about 2–3 wk, but are not optimal until after 6 wk

                (a) Warn of skin irritation and photosensitivity

          g. **Combination therapy** with diferent topical treatments

B. For **more severe acne** or if treatments listed above fail, consider adding to above treatment or substituting

      1. Oral antibiotics (titrate down to lowest effective dose once acne under control)

          a. Tetracycline: 500 mg b.i.d. to start, decreasing to 250 mg b.i.d. once acne controlled, decreasing to 125 mg for maintenance therapy

          b. Minocycline: 50–100 mg b.i.d.

          c. Trimethoprim/sulfamethoxazole: 80/400 mg b.i.d. to 160/800 mg b.i.d.

          d. Erythromycin: 250–500 b.i.d.

C. For **severe, disfiguring acne,** resistant to other therapies
   1. Oral isotretinoin (Accutane)
      a. This is a **teratogenic** drug
   2. **In women of childbearing age the following strict guidelines must be met before prescribing isotretinoin**
      a. Written, informed consent to use of drug
      b. Highly effective contraception or abstinence
      c. **Negative serum pregnancy test** within 2 wk
      d. Therapy begins 2–3 d after menses
      e. Patient must be told to read drug instructions
      f. Monitor monthly with serum pregnancy tests
      g. **Maximum single treatment course is 20 wk**
      h. Contraception or abstinence must continue after completion of course for 1 mo, with serum pregnancy test at end of that time
   3. Dosage
      a. Initial dose: 0.5–1 mg/kg in 2 divided doses
      b. Maximum dosage: 2 mg/kg daily
   4. Monitor LFTs monthly
   5. Other treatments (consult dermatologist for details)
      a. Corticosteroids (oral and intralesional)
      b. Oral contraceptives (women only)
      c. Antiandrogen
      d. Superficial exfoliation
      e. Dermabrasion and surgical treatments

IV. **Referral to Dermatologist is Often Helpful for**

A. Uncertainty of diagnosis or treatment
B. Recalcitrant acne or severe disease
C. Advice about a therapy or using combination therapies
D. Starting or follow-up for isotretinoin use

References

1. American Academy of Dermatology: Guidelines of care for acne vulgaris. J Am Acad Dermatol 22:676–680, 1990.
2. Leyden JJ, Shalita AR: Rational therapy for acne vulgaris: An update on topical treatment. J Am Acad Dermatol 15:907–915, 1986.

Adrenal Mass

I. **General Principles**

A. Prevalence of incidental adrenal mass is estimated at about 1–2%
B. Even with the presence of an incidental mass, prevalence of disease is extremely low, with the following estimates of prevalence

      1. Pheochromocytoma   6.5%
      2. Aldosteronoma   7.0%
      3. Glucocorticoid-secreting 0.035%
      4. Carcinoma   0.058%
      5. Prevalence is even lower when symptoms and signs are absent
  C. The low prevalence of these diseases exposes patients to a significant risk of false-negative or false-positive tests

II. Diagnostics

  A. **History and physical exam should seek symptoms and signs** of the above diseases
  B. **Laboratory data**
    1. Screening in asymptomatic persons with masses <6 cm
      a. Screen for pheochromocytoma with 24-hr urine for VMA, metanephrines, or catecholamines
      b. In **hypertensive patients,** screen for hyperaldosteronoma by serum potassium
      c. If clinical evaluation suggests excess glucocorticoids (Cushing's syndrome), consider either
        i. 24-hr urinary free cortisol level
        ii. Overnight dexamethasone suppression test
      d. If clinical evaluation suggests excess androgens (hirsutism or virilization)
        • See chapter on "Hirsutism"

III. Management

  A. General approach to **asymptomatic masses**
    1. Incidental masses ≥6 cm: refer for **excision**
    2. Incidental masses <**6 cm** with **negative screening tests**
      a. Monitor size with abdominal **CT scan at 3 mo**
        i. If enlarging, refer for excision
        ii. If stable, monitor again with CT scan at 6 or 12 mo and then periodically (e.g., yearly)
  B. If review of radiologic characteristics of the mass supports **suspicion of malignancy (e.g., irregularity, calcifications)**
    1. Refer for excision
  C. If **any of above tests are positive**
    1. Consult with or refer to endocrinologist for further evaluation
  D. If patient begins to have **symptoms of any adrenal disease**
    1. Investigate for suspected disease and/or refer
  E. **Alternative approach**
    1. Some practitioners recommend a more extensive evaluation of all masses, no matter what the size, and removal if >3 cm

IV. Referral to an Endocrinologist for

  A. Uncertainty of diagnosis or management
  B. Massess increasing in size

C. Suspected endocrinologic disorders
D. Urgent evaluation if carcinoma is suspected

Reference

Ross N, Aron D: Hormonal evaluation of the patient with an incidentally discovered adrenal mass. N Engl J Med 323:1401–1405, 1990.

Alcohol Abuse

I. General Principles

A. The earlier the diagnosis, the better the prognosis
B. Alcohol dependence is often associated with denial of the problem
C. Estimated prevalence in U.S.: 10–16% in general population
D. Alcoholism is associated with numerous familial psychiatric morbidities
E. The diagnosis of alcohol abuse or dependence is often missed because physicians shy away from stigmatization of patients, especially those in the same socioeconomic class
F. Be open and nonjudgmental; your help may save lives
G. **History and physical exam are often without significant abnormalities**
H. Alcohol abuse is a cause of secondary hypertension

II. Diagnostics

A. **History**
1. Family history: often positive for alcohol abuse or abstinence
2. GI complaints: vomiting, diarrhea, dyspepsia, gastritis
3. Onset or worsening of hypertension or arrhythmias
4. Accidents: car accidents, frequent minor trauma
5. Past or present legal or medical consequences of drinking
6. Duration of drinking problem
7. Amount, type of alcohol used, duration of use, binge behavior, and previous treatments
8. Effect on social life, work, and family life
9. Mood changes, behavioral changes
10. Sleep or sexual disturbances
11. Other drug or substance abuse

B. **Examination**
1. Vital signs: hypertension
2. Smell of alcohol on breath
3. State of dress and mental status
4. Evaluation of alcohol-associated disease: e.g., testicular atrophy, gynecomastia, palmar erythema, more than 5 spider nevi on upper body

C. **Screening**
  1. **The CAGE Questions**
     a. Have you felt that you should **C**ut down on your drinking?
     b. Do people **A**nnoy you by criticizing your drinking?
     c. Do you ever feel **G**uilty about drinking?
     d. Do you ever drink an **E**ye-opener?
  2. Likelihood ratios for positive answers to CAGE questions

Number of yeses	Likelihood ratio
3 or 4	250
2	7
1	1.3
0	0.2

  3. For details on how to use likelihood ratios, see chapter on "Diagnostic Decision-making"

D. **Laboratory data**
  1. **Not necessary for diagnosis or monitoring** (but may be helpful at times, especially if patient denies problem)
     a. CBC for MCV elevation (poor sensitivity)
     b. Aminotransferases and liver function tests
        i. AST (SGOT) rise more than twice ALT (SGPT) is suggestive of chronic alcohol use
        ii. GGT, alkaline phosphatase, bilirubin, and/or PT may also be elevated
     c. **Serum ETOH:** the following suggest chronic heavy ETOH use
        i. Level ≥**300 mg/dl at any time**
        ii. Level ≥**100 mg/dl at time of clinic visit**
        iii. Level ≥**150 mg/dl without signs of intoxication**

III. **Management and Treatment Options**

A. **Outpatient**
  1. Many phone directories have listings under Community Services, including
     a. Veterans' centers
     b. Alcoholics Anonymous (AA)
     c. Private care facilities
     d. Mental health clinics
  2. Drug treatment **(short term only, if used at all)**
     a. Benzodiazepines
        i. 1-week taper if patient likely to suffer alcohol withdrawal
     b. Vitamins: multivitamin q.d. or 1 wk of folate (1 mg) and thiamine (100 mg) q.d.
     c. Disulfiram (Antabuse): 125–500 mg q.d.
        i. Maximum dose: 500 mg q.d.

ii. If used, patient must
   (a) **Want** to comply with medication
   (b) **Understand** risk of drinking
   (c) Be **alcohol free** at time of therapy
   (d) Be **closely monitored**
   (e) Have **coincident counseling** and/or rehab therapy
iii. **Warn about alcohol in**
   (a) Cough syrups and mouthwashes
   (b) Alcohol-based sauces, cakes, foods
iv. Disulfiram also may interact with
   (a) Warfarin
   (b) Phenytoin
   (c) Metronidazole
   (d) Chlorpropamide
v. Can call Ayerst Laboratories for pamphlet, *Guidelines for Antabuse Users*

B. **Inpatient care**
   1. Consult local programs for availability
   2. Can improve 1-yr abstinence rates for selected alcoholics
   3. Advantages
      a. Removal from source of alcohol
      b. Observations during withdrawal
      c. Intensive psychological support

C. **Consider**
   1. Family members may need counseling or other support
      a. Self-help booklets
      b. Al-Anon
      c. Al-Ateen

References

1. American College of Physicians: Chemical dependence: A position paper. Am Coll Phys September, 1984.
2. Disulfiram treatment of alcoholism: Ann Intern Med 111:943–945, 1989.
3. Hays TJ, Spickard WA: Alcoholism: Early diagnosis and intervention. J Gen Intern Med 2:420–427, 1987.
4. Sackett DL, Hayes RB, Guyatt GH, Tugwell P: Clinical Epidemiology: A Basic Science for Clinical Medicine, 2nd ed. Boston, Little, Brown & Co., 1991.

Amenorrrhea

I. Definitions

A. **Primary amenorrhea:** absence of menarche by age 16 y/o
B. **Secondary amenorrhea:** absence of menses for 6 mo in women who have had prior menstrual periods

II. **General Principles**

    A. The average menstrual cycle is 28 d with a normal range of 18–40 d

    B. Physiologic amenorrhea occurs with pregnancy and frequently with lactation

    C. Prolonged periods of amenorrhea in a woman with normal circulating estrogens (e.g., polycystic ovaries) predisposes to endometrial hyperplasia

    D. Primary amenorrhea is usually caused by congenital abnormalities (e.g., intrauterine adhesions [Ashman's syndrome], imperforate hymen, pseudohermaphroditism)

    E. Estimated prevalence of nonphysiologic amenorrhea is 5%

    F. Other causes of secondary amenorrhea

        1. Anatomic

            a. Cervical stenosis after abortion

        2. Ovarian failure (with low circulating estrogens)

            a. Menopause

            b. Chemotherapy effects

            c. Premature ovarian failure

        3. Endocrine abnormalities

            a. Hypothalamic (with low circulating estrogens)

                i. Anorexia and bulimia

                ii. Exercise-induced

                iii. Severe systemic illnesses

            b. Hyperprolactinemia (pituitary microadenoma)

            c. Adrenal disorder/tumor

            d. Thyroid disease (normal circulating estrogens)

            e. Anovulation

                i. Polycystic ovarian syndrome (normal circulating estrogens)

        4. Drugs and medications

            a. Birth control pill-induced amenorrhea

            b. Post-birth control pill amenorrhea

            c. Phenothiazines

            d. Anabolic steroids

III. **Diagnostics**

    A. **History**

        1. Gynecologic and reproductive history

            a. Age at menarche

            b. Regularity of menstrual cycle prior to amenorrhea

            c. Last regular menstrual period

            d. Symptoms of menopause

            e. Hot flashes

            f. Night sweats

            g. Lack of vaginal lubrication

        2. Dietary habits and exercise

        3. Recent weight loss or life stressors

   4. Symptoms of hirsutism and virilization (rarely seen)
   5. Family history of premature ovarian failure
   6. Drugs and medications
   7. Galactorrhea
   8. Previous surgical and medical history
B. **Examination**
   1. Sexual history (e.g., pregnancy)
   2. Primary sexual characteristics (usually normal in secondary amenorrhea)
      a. Sexual development (see Tanner scales, Appendix 2)
      b. Breast development
      c. Body dimensions
   3. Galactorrhea
   4. Signs of hirsutism
      a. Abnormal hair patterns, including location of hair
   5. Signs of virilization
      a. Increased acne and temporal baldness
      b. Cliteromegaly
      c. Change in body habitus
   6. Evidence of anorexia nervosa, including body habitus and lanugo hair
   7. Pelvic examination for
      a. External genitalia (cliteromegaly)
      b. Aplasia of vagina or uterus
      c. Imperforate hymen
C. **Laboratory data**
   1. **Initial investigations for secondary amenorrhea**
      a. Urine pregnancy test
      b. Serum estradiol levels (for level of circulating estrogens)
      c. Prolactin
      d. TSH, FTI, or FT4
   2. **Further investigations for selected patients**
      a. If estradiol is low (indicating decreased ovarian function)
         i. FSH (LH is optional)
            (a) Decreased FSH is consistent with systemic illness, anorexia, and overexercise
            (b) Increased FSH >40 IU/ml is consistent with menopause and premature ovarian failure
            (c) An LH:FSH ratio >3:1 is consistent with polycystic ovaries
      b. If patient is hirsute or virilized, request DHEA-S and total testosterone levels
         i. Consider evaluation for androgen-secreting tumor if
            (a) DHEA-S >7.0 μg/dl
               or
            (b) Testosterone >200 ng/ml
      c. If clinical evaluation suggests Cushing's syndrome, consider

      i. 24-hr urine for free cortisol levels
     ii. Overnight dexamethasone suppression test

3. **Monitoring**
  a. **If prolactin level >20 ng/ml and TSH normal**
    i. Patient may have pituitary microadenoma
    ii. Measure **fasting** prolactin to confirm elevated prolactin; if still elevated
      (a) Consult with endocrinologist for appropriate tests
      (b) Check visual fields
  b. Women with premature ovarian failure should be evaluated for other autoimmune phenomena (e.g., autoimmune thyroid disease, diabetes) by an endocrinologist or gynecologic endocrinologist

IV. **Management**
  A. Evaluate patient clinically and with initial investigations
  B. Use results to refer patient for more specific evaluation or treatment
  C. Specific management should be undertaken under consultation with or by referral to specialist (gynecologist or endocrinologist)
  D. **Note:** once a woman becomes ovulatory, she needs contraception if pregnancy is not desired

V. **Referral for**
  A. Uncertainty of diagnostic protocol or management
  B. Specific treatment and monitoring
  C. Further evaluation once initial investigations requested

Reference

American College of Obstetricians and Gynecologists: Amenorrhea. Am Coll Obstet Gynecol Tech Bull 128, May 1989.

Anemia

I. **Definition**

Anemia refers to a reduction in hemoglobin concentration

II. **General Principles**

  A. **Common causes of anemia** in the U.S.
    1. Iron deficiency
    2. Thalassemia
    3. Chronic inflammatory, infectious, or malignant diseases
    4. Sickle-cell disease

5. B$_{12}$ or folate deficiency
6. Primary bone marrow disease (myelodysplasia, leukemia)
7. Toxins, such as alcohol

B. **Classifications of anemia** are frequently based on
   1. **Mean corpuscular volume** (MCV)
      a. MCV reflects average volume of the red cells over previous 120 d
   2. **Red blood cell distribution width** (RDW)
      a. RDW measures the degree of variations in red cell volumes at a given point in time
   3. **Reticulocyte count** (RC)
      a. Quantifies the number of young red cells in the peripheral circulation at a given point in time
      b. Helps differentiate hemolysis or acute blood loss from hypoplastic, hypoproliferative anemia
   4. **Corrected reticulocyte count** (CRC)
      a. CRC = RC × patient's hematocrit/normal hematocrit
   5. **Red cell characteristics on blood smear**
      a. **Size:** microcytic, macrocytic, or normocytic
      b. **Staining:** hypochromic, normochromic
      c. **Shape:** spherocytic, sickle

C. **Abnormalities and associated disorders**
   1. **Target cells**
      a. Iron deficiency
      b. Thalassemia
      c. Sickle cell disease
      d. Hemoglobin C disease
      e. Liver disease
      f. Splenectomy or hyposplenism
   2. **Anisocytosis** (red cell size differences)
      a. Iron deficiency anemia
      b. Sideroblastic anemia
   3. **Poikilocytosis** (red cell shape differences)
      a. Fe deficiency
      b. Thalassemia (teardrop poikilocytosis)
      c. Myelofibrosis (teardrop poikilocytosis)
   4. **Hypersegmented neutrophils/megaloblasts**
      a. B$_{12}$ deficiency
      b. Folate deficiency
   5. **Basophilic stippling**
      a. Lead poisoning
      b. Thalassemia
      c. Significant hemolysis
   6. **Sickle cells**
      a. Sickle-cell anemias
   7. **Sphereocytes**
      a. Hereditary spherocytosis
      b. Autoimmune hemolytic anemia
      c. Cold agglutinins

8. **Red cell fragments**
    a. Intravascular hemolysis
        i. Paroxysmal nocturnal hemoglobinuria
        ii. Artificial cardiac valves or any fragmentation hemolysis
        iii. Thrombotic thrombocytopenic purpura
9. **Heinz bodies**
    a. G6PD disease
    b. Thalassemias
    c. Other hemoglobinopathies
    d. Splenectomy

D. **Bone marrow aspiration and biopsy** are used to describe
    1. Cellularity and maturation
    2. Architecture of bone marrow
    3. Presence of abnormal cells
    4. Presence of iron stores
    5. Presence of megakaryocytes

III. **Diagnostics**

A. **History**
    1. **Presence of symptoms of anemia**
        a. Dyspnea, palpitations, angina, syncopal episodes
        b. Fatigue and weakness
        c. Headache, lightheadedness, difficulty concentrating
        d. Nausea, indigestion
        e. Sore tongue or mouth
        f. Pica
        g. Progressive dementia or confusion
    2. Back or bony pains
    3. History of frequent gallstones
    4. Family history: genetic heritage, anemias, splenectomy
    5. Medications such as AZT
    6. HIV risk factors, when appropriate
    7. Alcohol use and dietary habits (e.g., strict vegetarianism)
    8. Cause(s) of blood loss or anemia
        a. Melena or blood in stool
        b. Menstrual history and heaviness of blood flow
        c. History of renal, endocrine, rheumatologic, or other chronic disease(s)
        d. History of valvular heart disease

B. **Examination**
    1. General appearance: pallor, sallowness of skin, jaundice
    2. General mental state for confusion, disorientation
    3. Tongue for glossitis
    4. Cardiac examination for murmur(s)
    5. Abdominal examination for splenomegaly, masses
    6. Neurologic examination for decreased position and vibration sense, reflexes, and plantar response

7. Rectal examination and fecal occult blood test (FOBT)
8. Fingernails for signs of Fe deficiency

C. **Laboratory data**
   1. **Initial investigations for detection and classification** of anemia
      a. Complete blood count and indices (including RDW)
      b. Blood smear
      c. Reticulocyte count
   2. **For selected patients,** depending on clinical and laboratory evaluation above
      a. **If reticulocyte count is significantly elevated,** consider hemolytic anemia
         i. Reexamine peripheral blood smear
         ii. Further data in support of hemolysis may include any of
            (a) LDH (elevated)
            (b) Total and (in)direct bilirubin (elevated)
            (c) Haptoglobin (decreased)
            (d) Urine hemosiderin (elevated in intravascular hemolysis)
               (i) Paroxysmal nocturnal hemoglobinuria
               (ii) Artificial cardiac valves
         iii. For detection of type of hemolysis, consider
            (a) Sickle-cell preparation for blood smear that indicates sickle cells
            (b) HB electrophoresis for suspected hemoglobinopathies
            (c) Coombs' test for autoimmune hemolysis
            (d) Red-cell enzyme tests for G6PD deficiency and other enzymopathies
            (e) Red-cell membrane tests
               (i) Osmotic fragility
                  • For hereditary spherocytosis
               (ii) Sucrose lysis
                  • For paroxysmal nocturnal hemoglobinuria
      b. **IF MCV is decreased and RDW is elevated,** consider iron deficiency
         i. Further data may include
            (a) Fe (low)
            (b) Total iron-binding capacity (TIBC) (elevated)
            (c) Iron saturation (ratio usually <15%), where the ratio = Fe/TIBC
         ii. Optional data
            (a) Ferritin (low)
               (i) Can be an acute-phase reactant and may be elevated in liver disease
               (ii) A costly test and not always needed for diagnosis

      iii. Early iron deficiency may present with normal MCV but elevated RDW

c. If MCV is decreased, RDW is normal, consider
    i. Thalassemia
      (a) Further data may include
        (i) Fe studies to exclude iron deficiency
        (ii) Hemoglobin (Hb) electrophoresis, which is usually normal in alpha-thalassemia
        (iii) Quantitative assay for HbA2, which is elevated in beta-thalassemia minor
        (iv) Heinz body prep for HbH disease
      (b) In severe thalassemia with significant anemia, RDW may be increased
    ii. Anemia of chronic disease
      (a) Diagnosis is primarily one of exclusion
      (b) Usually associated with inflammatory disorders (such as connective tissue disease), malignancy, HIV, renal insufficiency

d. If MCV and RDW are normal, consider
    i. Recent hemorrhage
      (a) Usually associated with increased reticulocyte count
      (b) Urgent investigation usually required
    ii. Hereditary spherocytosis
      (a) Further data may include
        (i) Blood smear
        (ii) Coombs' test
        (iii) Osmotic fragility
    iii. Anemia of chronic disease usually has normal MCV and RDW
    iv. Endocrinopathies (e.g., thyroid disorder)
    v. Sideroblastic anemia

e. If MCV is normal and RDW elevated, consider
    i. Early Fe deficiency
    ii. Hemoglobinopathies
      (a) Further data may include
        (i) HB electrophoresis
        (ii) Red-cell membrane tests
    iii. Myelofibrosis
      (a) Further data may include bone marrow examination
    iv. Liver disease
    v. Renal insufficiency (uremia)

f. If MCV and RDW are elevated, consider
    i. **B_{12} or folate deficiency**
      (a) Further data may include
        (i) Blood smear for hypersegmented neutrophils
        (ii) RBC folate or serum folate
        (iii) Serum B_{12}

    ii. Autoimmune hemolytic anemia
      (a) Further data may include
        (i) Reticulocyte count
        (ii) LDH, bilirubin, and haptoglobin
        (iii) Coombs' test
        (iv) Blood smear for spherocytes
    iii. Toxins such as alcohol (see below)
    iv. Cold agglutinin disease
    v. Liver disease
    vi. Renal insufficiency (uremia)

  g. If MCV elevated and RDW normal, consider
    i. Alcohol abuse
      (a) Further data may include
        (i) Folate and B_{12} levels as above
        (ii) Evaluation for alcohol dependency
    ii. Thyroid disorders
      (a) Further data may include
        (i) B_{12} and folate levels as above
        (ii) FT4 and TSH
    iii. AZT treatment in HIV disease

3. **Indications for a bone marrow examination**
  a. Supportive evidence for a suspected anemia
  b. Anemia not diagnosed by above studies
  c. Anemia refractory to treatment
  d. Suspected myelofibrosis, myelodysplasia, aplastic anemia, sideroblastic anemia
  e. Suspected infiltrative disease: malignancy, granulomas, infectious diseases
  f. To confirm early Fe deficiency when MCV is not decreased and/or Fe studies are equivocal

IV. Management

A. General approach

1. **Treat anemia** when available treatment exists
  a. If vitamin deficiency: treat with appropriate replacement therapy
  b. Consider erythropoietin therapy
    i. If patient has anemia because of renal dysfunction
    ii. If patient has zidovudine-associated anemia and serum erythropoietin is < 500 U/ml
  c. **Transfusion is considered if** patient has
    i. Acute symptomatic anemia
      (a) Urgent hospital evaluation and treatment required
    ii. Chronic anemia with the following symptoms
      (a) Syncope
      (b) Dyspnea
      (c) Angina

        (d) Postural hypotension
        (e) Cerebrovascular symptoms: TIAs
- d. **Transfusions should not be used**
  - i. For enhancement of feeling of well-being
  - ii. In absence of symptoms listed above
  - iii. As a substitute for above treatments

2. **Evaluate underlying cause for**
   - a. Iron deficiency anemia
   - b. B_{12} deficiency
   - c. Refractory anemias
   - d. Undiagnosed anemias
   - e. Suspected malignant or aplastic disease
   - f. Suspected infiltrative disease

3. **Monitor response to therapy**
   - a. Usual markers include
     - i. Clinical evaluation for symptoms and general sense of well-being
     - ii. CBC and indices (including RDW)
     - iii. Reticulocyte count

B. **Specific anemias**
   1. **Iron deficiency anemia**
      - a. Evaluation
        - i. Unless patient has obvious cause of deficiency (e.g., menorrhagia, recent blood loss)
          - (a) Evaluate lower GI tract by either
            - (i) Colonscopy
              or
            - (ii) Sigmoidoscopy and double-contrast barium enema
          - (b) Evalute upper GI tract by either upper GI barium series or endoscopy
      - b. **Treatment**
        - i. $FeSO_4$: 325 mg orally t.i.d.
        - ii. Continue for 3–6 mo after hematocrit normalizes
          - (a) Consider starting q.d. or b.i.d. dose and titrating upward to t.i.d. to minimize GI upset
          - (b) Warn patient to expect change in stool consistency and color and, occasionally, change in bowel habit (diarrhea or constipation)
      - c. **Monitoring**
        - i. Evaluate within 3–4 wk
          - (a) Clinical examination
          - (b) CBC, which rises at about 1 g/2–4 wk
          - (c) Reticulocytes, which may be slightly elevated
        - ii. If CBC and/or reticulocyte shows response
          - (a) Reevaluate periodically until hematocrit normalizes
        - iii. If no response is seen, consider

          (a) Noncompliance with therapy
          (b) Refractory anemia

2. **Folate deficiency**
   a. **Treatment**
      i. Folate 1 mg PO q.d.
      ii. Anemia often resolves within 8–12 wk
   b. **Evaluation**
      i. Further evaluation should be undertaken if
         (a) Evidence suggests underlying chronic hemolysis
         (b) Alcoholism is likely
   c. **Monitoring**
      i. Clinical and marrow response should occur within 1–2 wk
      ii. Advise patient that diet should include fresh fruits and vegetables
      iii. Daily folate supplement is considered for
         (a) Chronic hemolytic states
         (b) Exfoliative skin diseases
         (c) Pregnant women
         (d) Certain medications, including methotrexate
         (e) Renal failure (sometimes)
         (f) Mechanical heart valves

3. **B_{12} deficiency**
   a. **Treatment**
      i. For patients with abnormal GI absorption: B_{12}, 1000 μg q mo IM
   b. **Further evaluation**
      i. Unless patient has obvious cause of deficiency (e.g., strict vegan vegetarianism, gastrectomy), consider evaluation for
         (a) Pernicious anemia
         (b) Blind loop syndrome
   c. **Monitoring**
      i. Clinical and marrow responses are usually seen with 1–2 wk
      ii. Patients with abnormal GI absorption need IM injections monthly for life

V. **Referrals to Hematologist Should Be Considered for**

A. Uncertainty of diagnosis or treatment
B. Undiagnosed or refractory anemias
C. Anemia with thrombocytopenia and/or leukopenia
D. Suspected hematologic deficiency
E. Suspected infiltrative disease
F. Suspected myelofibrosis, aplastic anemia, myelodysplasia, or other serious underlying marrow disorder

References

Author's note: A search of the published literature did not reveal comprehensive, contemporary guidelines, reviews, or prospectively determined protocols for evaluation of anemia. The chapter above has been compiled from the following:

1. American College of Physicians: Practice strategies for elective red blood cell transfusion. Ann Intern Med 116:403–406, 1992.
2. Bergin JJ: Evaluation of anemia: Getting the most out of the MCV, RDW, and other tests. Postgrad Med 77:253–269, 1985.
3. Beutler E: The common anemias. JAMA 259:2433–2437, 1988.
4. Djulbegovic B, Hadley T, Pasic R: A new algorithm for diagnosis of anemia. Postgrad Med 85:119–130, 1989.
5. Karnard A, Poskitt TR: The automated complete blood count. Arch Intern Med 1270–1272, 1985.

Supplementary data from:
1. Current Medical Diagnosis and Treatment. Norwalk, CT, Appleton & Lange, 1990, pp 328–345.
2. Harrison's Principles of Internal Medicine, 12th ed. New York, McGraw-Hill, 1991, pp 344–348.

Asthma

I. Definition

A. Asthma is characterized by bronchospasm, causing any or all of:
   1. Dyspnea
   2. Wheezing
   3. Cough

II. General Principles

A. Asthma afflicts up to 5% of the U.S. population
B. Presentation may be of chronic nonproductive and/or nocturnal cough

III. Diagnostics

A. **History**
   1. Symptoms: episodic wheeze, cough, dyspnea
   2. Age at onset
   3. How often attacks occur
   4. Previous hospitalizations and intubations
   5. Prior and present treatment and medications
   6. Stimuli that precipitate attacks
      a. Dust and environmental allergens
      b. Occupational exposure
      c. Exercise
      d. Cold air

      e. Drugs: aspirin (NSAIDs), beta blockers
      f. Foods or beverages
    7. Family history of atopy, allergic disease
    8. Personal history of allergic disease: rhinitis, sinusitis, conjunctivitis, postnasal drip, nasal polyps

B. **Examination** (under nonacute circumstances)
    1. Eyes, ears, nose, and throat: signs of allergic disease and/or nasal polyps
    2. Respiratory examination, including forced expiration maneuver to manifest end-expiratory wheeze

C. **Laboratory data**
    1. For diagnosis, quantification of severity, and/or monitoring
      a. Peak flow meter at baseline examination and for quantifying over time the severity of disease
      b. Spirometric studies and peak flow measurements may indicate
        i. Reduced FEV_1 and peak flow rate
        ii. Reduced FEV_1/FVC ratio
        iii. Increase of $>15\%$ with bronchodilator
      c. CBC with differential
        i. Eosinophilia is common in asthmatics
          (a) If $>3,000/mm^3$ and leukocytosis, consider
            (i) Hypereosinophilic syndrome
            (ii) Loffler's syndrome
            (iii) Allergic aspergillosis
            (iv) Churg-Strauss granulomatosis
      d. Chest x-ray
        i. Occasionally helpful in diagnosis of asthma (e.g., hyperinflation of lung fields)
        ii. Mostly used for acute severe asthma
      e. Arterial blood gases
        i. Usually reserved for acute severe asthma
      f. Bronchial provocation tests are used for diagnosis of suspected asthma in a currently asymptomatic person and in suspected occupational asthma
        i. Refer to pulmonary consultant for provocation testing
    2. **For selected patients**
      a. If history suggests allergic stimuli, consider
        i. Paranasal x-ray for sinusitis
        ii. Skin tests: prick, scratch, or intradermal
        iii. Radioallergosorbent test (RAST): in vitro test (detects antigen-specific IgE antibodies)

IV. **Management**

A. **Attempt to reduce exposure** to specific stimuli, when known, that provoke asthmatic attack
    1. Animal dander
    2. House dust mite
    3. Cold temperatures

B. **Pharmacologic therapy**
   1. **Beta-adrenergic agonists**, usually prescribed as metered-dose inhalers (MDI)
      a. As needed up to 2 puffs every 4–6 hr, up to 12 puffs daily
         i. Medium-acting preparations
            (a) Metaproterenol (Alupent)
         ii. Long-acting preparations
            (a) Albuterol (Proventil, Ventolin)
            (b) Terbutaline (Bricanyl)
      b. Patients need careful instruction on proper use of an MDI
         i. If patient has difficulty with MDI, try a **spacer** such as Inspirease
      c. For exercise-induced asthma take 2 puffs of beta agonist 30 min before exercise
   2. **Corticosteroids** (inhaled or oral)
      a. Acute exacerbations may benefit from short course of oral steroids, especially if
         i. Cough and wheeze have lasted >48 hr without treatment
         ii. Patient has had frequent attacks recently
         iii. Recent attacks have required oral steroids
      b. Usual dose of oral prednisone is 40 mg q.d. or equivalent
      c. Try to taper off oral steroids within 2 wk
      d. Inhaled steroids may help reduce frequent attacks and are receiving more attention as frontline drugs for reduction of bronchospastic events
         i. Usual dose is 2 puffs q.i.d. or equivalent
         ii. Take after using bronchodilator
         iii. Maximum dosage is 16 puffs daily
         iv. May be started while patient tapers off oral dose
         v. Rinse mouth and throat after use to reduce risk for oral candidiasis
      e. Preparations of inhaled steroids
         i. Azmacort: triamcinolone acetonide
         ii. Vanceril and Beclovent: beclomethasone dipropionate
   3. **Ipratropium bromide** (Atrovent)
      a. Useful in some asthmatics
      b. Can try alone or with beta agonists
      c. Usual dose is 2 puffs of MDI aerosol q.i.d.
      d. Maximum dose is 12 puffs per 24 hr
   4. **Theophylline**
      a. Use is controversial, but theophylline may help control frequent attacks when bronchodilators and other therapies are inadequate
      b. Monitor level soon after starting drug (e.g., 1 wk)
      c. Initial dose is usually 200–300 mg b.i.d.

      d. Drug preparations are not interchangeable
      e. Serum levels may increase if taken in conjunction with
         i. Cimetidine
         ii. Allopurinol
         iii. Erythromycin
      f. Serum levels may decrease if taken in conjunction with
         i. Cigarette smoking
         ii. Phenytoin
         iii. Rifampicin
      g. Toxic symptoms may occur within therapeutic levels (10–20 μg/ml)
         i. Nervousness and tremor
         ii. GI symptoms
         iii. Arrhythmias and seizures

   5. **Cromolyn**
      a. In suspected allergy-mediated asthma consider 4–6-wk trial of therapy to determine if successful
      b. Dose is 2 puffs q.i.d.
      c. For exercise-induced bronchospasm take 2 puffs 10–15 min prior to exercise

   6. **Immunotherapy**
      a. Refer to allergist/immunologist

C. **Nonpharmacologic therapies**
   1. Smoking cessation should be emphasized
   2. Vaccinations
      a. Influenza: yearly for those with COPD/asthma
      b. Pneumococcal: for those >50 y/o with COPD/asthma

V. **Referral to Pulmonologist for**

A. Uncertainty of diagnosis or treatment
B. Bronchoprovocation or allergy testing
C. If ENT abnormality suspected
D. Moderate to severe asthmatics with frequent attacks
E. Poor response to simple standard therapies
F. For immunotherapy, when necessary

References

1. American Thoracic Society: Standards for the diagnosis and care of patients with chronic obstructive pulmonary disease (COPD) and asthma. Am Rev Respir Dis 136:225–243, 1987.
2. National Institutes of Health: Guidelines for the Diagnosis and Management of Asthma. DHHS No. 91-304A, 1991.

Atrial Fibrillation

I. **General Principles**
   A. Prevalence of atrial fibrillation (AF): 2% in general population; 5% in persons > 60 y/o
   B. Associated with 50% of cardioembolic strokes
   C. Conditions associated with atrial fibrillation include but are not limited to
      1. Nonvalvular heart disease (70% of cases), including
         a. Coronary artery disease
         b. Hypertension
      2. Valvular heart disease
         a. Rheumatic mitral disease
      3. Pulmonary emboli (2.5%)
      4. Thyrotoxicosis (1%)
   D. Stroke rate is estimated at
      1. 5% per year in persons with nonvalvular AF and coexisting cardiovascular disease
      2. >5% with valvular atrial fibrillation
      3. <0.5% per year in persons <60 y/o without evidence of coexisting cardiovascular disease ("lone" atrial fibrillation)

II. **Diagnostics**
   A. **History and examination** for atrial fibrillation are oriented to determining
      1. Hemodynamic stability
      2. Time of onset of atrial fibrillation
      3. Possible underlying causes
   B. **Laboratory data**
      1. EKG
      2. CBC
      3. PT, PTT (prior to beginning anticoagulation)
      4. Electrolytes, creatinine, BUN
      5. Metabolites: calcium, phosphorus, magnesium
      6. Thyroid function tests: TSH, FT4 or FTI
      7. CXR
      8. Echocardiography
         a. Transthoracic
         b. Esophageal (recommended by some practitioners)

III. **Management**
   A. **General approach**
      1. Management consists of rate control and, whenever possible, cardioversion
      2. If patient is not a candidate for cardioversion, or if cardioversion fails, long-term anticoagulaton may be appropriate

B. **Anticoagulation in persons with stable atrial fibrillation**
  1. The following patients should be anticoagulated if no exclusion criteria apply
     a. Patients with AF secondary to valvular heart disease
     b. Older patients (>60 y/o) with nonvalvular AF
  2. Controversy regards anticoagulation for
     a. Lone AF and person <60 y/o
     b. Paroxysmal AF
  3. Exclusion criteria for anticoagulation
     a. Bleeding disorders
     b. Previous hemorrhage
     c. Active peptic ulcer disease
     d. Alcoholism
     e. Uncontrolled HTN
     f. Gait disorders
     g. Severe renal or liver disease
     h. Noncompliance
C. **Dosage and monitoring**
  1. For valvular AF and nonvalvular AF (patient >60 y/o)
     a. Start warfarin at 4–5 mg q.d., check PT 4–6 d later, and monitor closely until PT stabilizes
     b. Increase PT to 1.3–1.5 × baseline value
     c. If patient is unable to use warfarin, consider aspirin: 325 mg q.d.
  2. For nonvalvular AF (lone AF and patient <60 y/o), consider aspirin: 325 mg q.d.

IV. **Referral to Cardiologist for**

  A. Uncertainty of diagnosis or treatment
  B. Cardioversion
  C. If questions arise on need to start or stop anticoagulation

Reference

For details concerning randomized controlled trials consult:
Conference: Stroke prevention in nonvalvular atrial fibrillation. Ann Intern Med 115:727–741, 1991.

B

Breast Lesions

I. **General Principles**

    A. **The incidence of breast cancer** is now about 180,000 per year

    B. **Survival at 5 years**
- 1. 85% for stage I
- 2. 66% for stage II
- 3. 41% for stage III
- 4. 10% for stage IV

    C. Lifetime probability for breast cancer is >7%

    D. Early detection lengthens lifespan and survival rates

    E. No test is perfect; lab and clinical conditions vary as do underlying chances for malignancy in a given individual

    F. **Risk of breast cancer** is associated with
- 1. Age
- 2. Previous history of cancerous breast lump
- 3. Higher socioeconomic status
- 4. Childbearing after age 30
- 5. Nulliparity
- 6. Obesity
- 7. Menarche prior to age 12
- 8. Menopause after age 53
- 9. First-degree relative(s) with breast cancer
- 10. Previous tissue diagnosis of ductal or lobular hyperplasia, with or without atypia

    G. Probability of cancerous lesions for a 40-year-old woman
- 1. If asymptomatic and without risk factors: 1%
- 2. With a palpable mass: 20%
- 3. With clinical signs of malignancy: 80%

    H. Accuracy of detection of cancer by mammogram in an asymptomatic woman
- 1. Sensitivity = 75% (66–94%)
- 2. Specificity = 90% (50–90%)
- 3. With a negative screening mammogram, probability of cancer is approximately 0.2%
- 4. With a positive screening mammogram, probablity of cancer is approximately 10%

    I. For **women with palpable masses,** accuracy of a mammogram in detecting cancer
- 1. Sensitivity = 80% (79–88%)
- 2. Specificity = 90% (85–93%)

II. **Recommendations for Screening**
  A. Screening is by monthly self breast exam and yearly breast exam (especially after age 35) by a physician
  B. Mammography is recommended as follows
    1. American College of Physicians
      a. Mammogram yearly from age 50, unless other risks noted
    2. American College of Radiology
      a. Mammogram yearly after age 40
      b. Baseline examination, 35–40 y/o
    3. American College of Obstetrics and Gynecology and the American Cancer Society
      a. Mammogram every 1–2 yr, 40–50 y/o
      b. Mammogram yearly after age 50
      c. Baseline examination, 35–40 y/o
        i. **Note:** ACOG mentions that for patients at higher risk, consider baseline at age 30

III. **Diagnostics**
  A. **History**
    1. Time since lump first noted
    2. Change in size of lump since first noted
    3. Nipple discharge
    4. Change in size in relation to menstrual cycle
    5. Tenderness
    6. Family history of breast cancer in first-degree relatives
    7. Contraceptive pill and/or other hormone use
    8. Systemic signs: weight loss, bone pain, fatigue
  B. **Examination**
    1. Visual examination of breast with patient sitting and lying down
    2. Characteristics of lump, including size, shape, contour, nodularity, color, attachment to soft tissues
    3. Retraction of skin around lump
    4. Presence of nipple discharge
    5. Lymph node enlargement in axillae and supraclavicular areas
  C. **Laboratory data**
    1. For suspicious area on mammography in woman without a palpable lump
      a. Further investigation must include
        i. Biopsy from area of suspicion, usually done at time of mammography
        ii. Further evaluation based on result of biopsy and mammogram
    2. **Imaging studies for a palpable breast lump**
      a. In a woman 35 y/o or older, or in a woman (20 y/o or older) with an increased risk for breast cancer or with a lesion suspicious for carcinoma
        i. Mammography **and**
        ii. Fine-needle aspiration (FNA)

b. In a woman <35 y/o with a suspected cystic mass
   i. Ultrasound scan of breast
      (a) If mass not cystic patient should have both
         (i) Mammography
         (ii) FNA or open biopsy
   ii. Fine-needle aspiration
      (a) For aspiration of suspected cyst
      (b) For cytology of mass or cyst
3. Further studies and monitoring
  a. FNA for cystic masses (as assessed by ultrasound) that persist
  b. **Referral for open biopsy is appropriate if**
    i. FNA reveals bloody cyst
    ii. Mass persists after aspiration
    iii. Mass continues to recur after 1 or 2 aspirations
    iv. Mass is solid and is not a fibroadenoma
    v. There is bloody nipple discharge or nipple ulceration
    vi. Clinical evaluation is suspicious for inflammatory breast carcinoma
4. **Note:** negative results on any study are insufficient when clinical evaluation suggests carcinoma
  a. Refer to surgeon or specialist
  b. **Note:** Some physicians (NEJM, 1992) advocate FNA for any palpable mass, followed by mammography for any woman 20 y/o or older and who is not pregnant, whether the mass is cystic or solid. Further management then depends on results of FNA and/or mammogram. In this diagnostic algorithm, ultrasound is not generally used.

IV. **Referral to Specialist Should be Considered for**

A. Further monitoring and/or management after initial evaluation and laboratory studies
B. Uncertainty of evaluation
C. Surgical intervention when appropriate

References

1. American College of Obstetrics and Gynecology: Nonmalignant conditions of the breast. ACOG Tech Bull No. 156, June, 1991.
2. American College of Obstetrics and Gynecology: Carcinoma of the breast. ACOG Tech Bull No. 158, August, 1991.
3. American College of Radiology: Policy statement: On sonography for the detection and diagnosis of breast disease. September, 1984.
4. Donegan WL: Evaluation of a palpable breast mass. N Engl J Med 327:937–942, 1992.
5. Health and Public Policy Committee, American College of Physicians: The use of diagnostic tests for screening and evaluating breast lesions. Ann Intern Med 103:143–146, 1985.
6. Mushlin AI: Diagnostic tests in breast cancer: Clinical strategies based on diagnostic probabilities. Ann Intern Med 103:79–85, 1985.

C

Carotid Stenosis and Bruits

I. **General Principles**

   A. Approximately 50–65% of patients with carotid stenosis have a carotid bruit

   B. Approximately 50–65% of patients with a cervical bruit noted on examination have carotid stenosis

   C. Bruits become audible when about 50% of the lumen is stenosed
      1. The higher the pitch, the tighter the stenosis
      2. Bruits that are high-pitched and fade into diastole are often hemodynamically important
      3. Stenosis >70% is considered hemodynamically important

   D. Emboli originating from the carotid bifurcation usually go to ophthalmic artery or middle or anterior cerebral artery territories

   E. Asymptomatic carotid bruit has approximately a 1–1.5% annual (ipsilateral) stroke risk in untreated patients

   F. The term ipsilateral TIA (or stroke) refers to neurologic changes corresponding to the ipsilateral carotid artery (e.g., a left carotid plaque causing symptoms associated with emboli to the left cerebral hemisphere)

II. **Diagnostics**

   A. **History**
      1. TIA symptoms in recent past (e.g., within past 4–6 mo)
         a. Number
         b. Description of neurologic symptoms
         c. Duration of events
      2. Ipsilateral amaurosis fugax symptoms
      3. Small ipsilateral stroke with good recovery
      4. Peripheral nervous system symptoms
      5. Other symptoms of peripheral vascular or coronary artery disease, such as angina or limb claudication
      6. Cardiovascular history (e.g., atrial fibrillation, MI, angina) and risk factors for coronary artery disease
      7. Smoking and alcohol history
      8. History of other diseases that may present similarly to TIAs
         a. Migraine
         b. Seizures
         c. Systemic diseases such as collagen vascular disease, malignancy, hematologic disorders (polycythemia vera, leukemia), and diabetes with hypoglycemic episodes

B. **Examination**
   1. Blood pressure in both arms
   2. Neck bruits
   3. Cardiac exam
   4. Abdominal exam for mass (AAA) and/or bruits
   5. Complete neurologic exam
   6. Peripheral vascular exam

C. **Laboratory data**
   1. **Initial investigations**
      a. CBC for anemia, polycythemia, or elevated white cell count
      b. EKG
      c. ESR (for evidence of vasculitis)
      d. Serum glucose (for evidence of diabetes)
      e. Creatinine and BUN
      f. Cholesterol and triglycerides
      g. Duplex scan (if available) or Doppler ultrasound of carotid arteries
   2. **Further investigations in selected patients**
      a. PT, PTT for patients suspected of having a coagulopathy or in patients who are to be anticoagulated
      b. Echocardiography for patients suspected of having cardiac disease
         i. Person under age 40 with history of stroke or TIAs
         ii. Persons with abnormal cardiac examination such as murmurs or cardiomegaly
         iii. Persons wih a history of MI, valvular disease, or atrial fibrillation
      c. CT scan of the brain, especially in persons with neurologic deficits

III. **Management**

A. **General approach for patient with cervical bruit**
   1. Can be divided into 3 categories
      a. Asymptomatic bruit with no stenosis
      b. Asymptomatic stenosis (with or without bruit)
      c. Symptomatic disease (with or without stenosis)
   2. Includes evaluation of all patients for cardiac risk factors (e.g., smoking, hyperlipidemia, diabetes, hypertension), with modifications made accordingly

B. **For asymptomatic bruits with no stenosis**
   1. Evaluate and modify cardiac risk factors
   2. Consider, if no contraindications, aspirin: 325 mg/d

C. **For asymptomatic stenosis with or without a bruit**
   1. Evaluate and modify cardiac risk factors
   2. Consider, if no contraindications, aspirin, 325 mg/d
   3. Surgery, although controversial, may be beneficial for
      a. High-grade stenosis (>70%) with or without other risk factors for stroke (e.g., hypertension, hyperlipidemia, smoking) and contralateral carotid artery occlusion

b. In the setting of CABG, endarterectomy can be performed as prophylaxis against stroke

D. **For symptomatic disease with or without a bruit**
  1. Evaluate and modify cardiac risk factors
  2. Begin initial investigations, as noted above, and refer to neurologist
  3. If a bruit is heard on auscultation, with neurologic symptoms consistent with an ipsilateral lesion, anticoagulation should begin with aspirin: 325–1300 mg/d (unless contraindicated or if patient is already on warfarin)
  4. If the patient is alrealdy on aspirin, discuss use of ticlopidine with neurologist

E. **Surgery**
  1. **Considered beneficial** with any of
     a. High-grade **ipsilateral** stenosis (70–99%)
     b. 50% or greater stenosis with a large carotid ulcer
     c. Small stroke associated with lesions listed above if surgery can be delayed for 1 mo
  2. **Controverisal but may be beneficial** with any of
     a. Recurrent or crescendo TIAs despite medical therapy in patients without significant stenosis but with large carotid artery ulcer
     b. Moderate (30–69%) ipsilateral stenosis in symptomatic patients
  3. **Not indicated** with any of
     a. Occluded vessel
     b. Mildly stenosed (0–29%) vessel
     c. High surgical risk, including
        i. Patient is poor surgical candidate
        ii. Surgical team has high complication rate
     d. Large, completed stroke or stroke in evolution
     e. Symptoms from vertebrobasilar distribution

F. **Categories of stenoses and summary of recommendations for symptomatic patients**

Degree of Stenosis		Recommendation
Mild:	**0–29%**	Endarterectomy not recommended
Moderate:	**30–69%**	No definite recommendations
Severe:	**70–99%**	Endarterectomy may be indicated in properly selected asymptomatic patients
Occluded:	**100%**	Endarterectomy contraindicated

G. If evaluation of carotid lesion indicates that surgery may be beneficial, then assess perioperative cardiac risk
  • See chapter on "Cardiac Risks of Noncardiac Surgery" for details

H. Surgery, when indicated, must expose patients to as little risk as possible; surgical complication rates of the surgical team must be lower than the following

      1. Surgical mortality for endarterectomies $<1\%$
      2. Stroke-related morbidity $<3\%$ in symptomatic patients
      3. Stroke-related morbidity $<2\%$ in asymptomatic patients

IV. Referral to Vascular Surgeon for Symptomatic Carotid Bruit when

   A. Duplex/Doppler findings indicate significant disease
   B. Patient consents to surgery
   C. Patient has acceptable surgical risk profile
   D. Mortality and morbidity data from the surgical team are low

References

1. American College of Physicians: Indications for carotid endarterectomy. Ann Intern Med 111:675–677, 1989.
2. Carotid endarterectomy: Specific therapy based on pathophysiology. N Engl J Med, August 15, 1991.

Cataracts

I. Definition

A cataract is a lens opacification

II. General Principles

   A. The prevalence of cataracts increases with age
      1. Up to 50% of persons 65–74 y/o may have cataracts
   B. Cataracts are a significant cause of visual disability and blindness
   C. **Indications for surgery**
      1. Impairment of desired lifestyle or occupation due to loss of visual acuity
      2. Significant impairment of vision not alleviated by corrective lenses
      3. Disabling glare from bright lights
      4. Visual impairment under conditions of dim lighting
      5. Double vision
      6. Significant differences in vision between left and right eyes
      7. Presence of other eye diseases that may impair vision
   D. **Contraindications to surgery**
      1. Patient refuses surgery or is unfit for surgery
      2. Irreversible visual impairment
      3. Patient has satisfactory visual function with corrective lenses
      4. Patient does not have significant impairment in his/her lifestyle
   E. **Surgical risks**
      1. Retinal detachment
      2. Macular edema
      3. Secondary glaucoma (rare)

    4. Hyphema or lens dislocation (rare)

    5. Endophthalmitis (rare)

III. **Diagnostics in Primary-care Setting**

  A. **History**

    1. Presence of visual changes

      a. Loss of acuity in normal light

      b. Decreased vision in dim light

      c. Inability to perform daily occupational or leisure activities

      d. Disabling glare from car headlights or from other bright lights

      e. Diplopia or polyopia

      f. Inability to obtain unrestricted driver's license because of visual impairment

      g. Prior impairment of vision in either eye

      h. History of glaucoma or other eye disease that may impair vision

  B. **Examination**

    1. Extraocular muscle movements

    2. Pupillary response to light

    3. Direct ophthalmoscopy

    4. Visual field testing

    5. Visual acuity

  C. **Laboratory data**

    1. No routine data necessary in primary care for diagnosis of cataract

IV. **Management**

  A. **For persons with visual acuity 20/40 or better in the affected eye**

    1. Risks may outweigh benefits from surgery

    2. Surgery should be considered only for significant visual disability that is due to the cataract

    3. Corrective lenses may satisfactorily improve vision

  B. **For persons with visual acuity 20/50 or worse in the affected eye**

    1. Surgery is indicated if there is significant visual impairment due to the cataract, as described above

    2. Evaluate surgical risk if patient and ophthalmologist agree on surgery

V. **Referral to Ophthalmologist for**

  A. Uncertainty of evaluation or treatment

  B. Best corrected vision is 20/40 or worse

  C. Other suspected or documented eye diseases

  D. Surgical intervention when indicated

Reference

American Academy of Ophthalmology: Preferred Practice Pattern. Cataract in the Otherwise Healthy Adult Eye. September, 1989.

Cholesterol and Lipids

I. **General Principles**
   A. A cholesterol level of
      1. <200 mg/dl is **desirable**
      2. 200–239 mg/dl is **borderline**
      3. >240 mg/dl is considered **high risk**
         a. This represents the beginning of the upper 25% of the U.S. population
   B. Diagnosis is usually based on finding 2 elevated nonfasting cholesterol levels, taken at least 2 mo apart
   C. Elevation or distortion of lipid profile may occur with
      1. Drugs such as thiazides, beta blockers, progestins, anabolic steroids
      2. Diseases including hypothyroidism, diabetes mellitus, nephrotic syndrome, and obstructive liver disease
   D. Recommendations are for persons up to 70 y/o
      1. For recommendations for adolescents (<20 y/o), see chapter on "Adolescent Medicine"
   E. **Further evaluation based on risk stratification**
      1. Persons with cholesterol
         a. >240 mg/dl are at high risk
         b. From 200–239 mg/dl
            i. And definite CAD are at high risk
            ii. And 2 or more cardiac risk factors are at high risk

II. **Diagnostics**

   A. **History**
      1. Definite coronary artery disease (CAD)
         a. Prior MI
         b. Known angina pectoris
      2. Cardiac risk factors
         a. Male gender
         b. Family history of myocardial infarct or sudden death in sibling or parent before age 55
         c. Diabetes mellitus
         d. Hypertension
         e. Cigarette smoking >10/d, **currently**
         f. Cerebrovascular or peripheral vascular disease
         g. Overweight by >30%
         h. HDL <35 mg/dl
      3. Medications
   B. **Examination**
      1. Cardiac examination
      2. Peripheral vascular and carotid evaluation
      3. Presence of xanthelasma, xanthomas, and/or arcus corneae

C. **Laboratory data**
   1. Initial investigation is a nonfasting cholesterol level
   2. Further investigations for selected patients
      a. Urinalysis looking for nephrotic syndrome
      b. Serum glucose for detection of diabetes
      c. Thyroid function tests (TSH, FTI or FT4) if clinical evaluation indicates hypothyroidism
      d. **For a nonfasting cholesterol that is borderline** (200–239 mg/dl) in patient with definite CAD or 2 or more CAD risk factors
      or
      e. Patient has cholesterol >240 mg/dl
         i. Get **fasting** (12-hr fast) lipid levels
         ii. **Note:** LDL levels can be calculated by the equation LDL = total cholesterol – HDL – triglycerides/5
            (a) Considered correct if triglycerides <400 mg/dl

III. **Management**

   A. **General advice for all patients**
      1. Reduce alcohol intake
      2. Stop smoking
      3. Exercise: 20 min of aerobic activity at least 3 d/wk
      4. Reduce saturated fats and substitute, if necessary, monosaturated and polyunsaturated fats
   B. **If nonfasting cholesterol is <200 mg/dl,** repeat nonfasting cholesterol in 5 yr and give dietary advice about decreasing saturated fat intake
   C. **If nonfasting cholesterol is borderline (200–239 mg/dl) with no other risks for CAD,** then give dietary advice and remeasure nonfasting cholesterol in 1 yr.
      1. If total cholesterol is still borderline, reiterate dietary advice and remeasure nonfasting total cholesterol annually
   D. **If nonfasting cholesterol is borderline (200–239 mg/dl) and patient has definite CAD or 2 or more CAD risk factors or if nonfasting cholesterol is >240 mg/dl,** then management is contingent upon LDL level
      1. If LDL is **<130 mg/dl**, patient is low risk
         a. Give dietary advice
         b. Remeasure nonfasting total cholesterol in 3–5 yr
      2. **If LDL is between 130–159 mg/dl,** patient is borderline risk
         a. If patient has <2 cardiac risk factors, give dietary advice and repeat nonfasting total cholesterol yearly
         b. If patient has **2 or more cardiac risk factors,** start phase I diet (see below) and recheck nonfasting cholesterol level within 3–6 mo
      3. If LDL is **>160 mg/dl,** patient is high risk
         a. Start phase I diet (see below)
         b. Recheck nonfasting cholesterol within 3–6 mo

    4. If LDL cholesterol is >**225 mg/dl,** patient is very high risk
       a. Start phase I diet
       b. Start lipid-lowering drug
       c. **Note:** some practitioners start immediate drug therapy
         if LDL is >190 mg/dl

IV. **Treatment Guidelines**
  A. **Dietary therapy: phase I and II**
    1. **Phase I diet**
      a. Decrease all fats to 30% of caloric intake daily and saturated fats to <10%
      b. Decrease cholesterol to <300 mg/d
      c. Consider referral to nutritionist or give patient a self-help pamphlet to assist with compliance
      d. Dietary advice may be reinforced if person who cooks for patient is given counseling on diet as well
    2. **Monitor phase I diet** by clinical and cholesterol evaluation at 6 wk and 3 mo
      a. If after 3 mo patient's LDL is <130 mg/dl (when he/she has CAD or 2 risk factors for CAD) or <160 mg/dl (when he/she has one or no CAD risk factors), then patient should be monitored for dietary compliance and cholesterol levels every 3 mo during the next year and then every 6 mo thereafter
    3. If LDL has not been reduced to the above levels at 3 mo, then start **phase II diet**
      a. Decrease saturated fats to <7% of diet and cholesterol to <200 mg/d
      b. Referral to a nutritionist is likely needed for assisting patient in complying with such a strict diet
      c. LDL levels are evaluated as above
      d. Failure to attain goals at 3 mo of phase II diet indicates need for drug therapy
    4. If patient cannot tolerate phase I or II diet and LDL is still elevated, start drug treatment
    5. **Note:** to reduce cost of monitoring, total cholesterol level rather than LDL may be used to monitor progress during diet or drug therapy. Total cholesterol level of 200 mg/dl is a proxy for an LDL level of 130 mg/dl. Total cholesterol level of 240 mg/dl approximates an LDL level of 160 mg/dl
  B. **Drug therapy**
    1. **For elevated cholesterol (total or LDL) without elevated triglycerides**
      a. **Cholestyramine**
        i. Start at 4 g (or 1 packet), q.d.–b.i.d.
        ii. Take 1 hr after meals
        iii. Mix powder with juice, water, or milk
        iv. Take other drugs 1 hr before or 4 hr after cholestyramine

    v. Titrate slowly upward to higher doses

    vi. Maintenance dose is often about 2 packages b.i.d. (or equivalent in grams)

    vii. Maximum dose: 24 g

    viii. **Warn** patient of bloating, flatulence, constipation, heartburn

    ix. Monitor for

      (a) GI side effects

      (b) Increased triglyceride levels

b. **Cholestipol**

    i. Start at 5 g b.i.d.

    ii. Take 1 hr after meals

    iii. Mix powder with juice, water, or milk

    iv. Take other drugs 1 hr before or 4 hr after cholestipol

    v. Titrate slowly upward as necessary

    vi. Maximum dose is 15 g b.i.d.

    vii. **Warn** patient of bloating, flatulence, heartburn, constipation

    viii. Monitor for

      (a) GI effects

      (b) Increased triglyceride levels

c. **Nicotinic acid (niacin)**

    i. Start at 50 to 100 mg t.i.d., titrating upward weekly as tolerated (Note: some patients may need to start at 100 mg q.d. in order to tolerate side effects)

or Niacin SR, 750 mg

    i. Start at 1 tablet q.d. (or ½ tablet b.i.d.), titrating upward by 1 tablet/wk as tolerated

    ii. Therapeutic dose of niacin is usually 3 g/d

    iii. Maximum dose is 9 g/d

    iv. Take dose with meals

    v. Flushing and pruritus can be minimized by aspirin, 325 mg, ½ hr before taking niacin (not usually necessary with SR tablets)

    vi. Monitor

      (a) Blood glucose, uric acid, LFTs at 3 mo when titrating dose and at 6–12 mo once dosage stable

      (b) LFTs when switching from immediate-release to sustained-release formulations

    vii. Use caution when prescribing nicotinic acid with

      (a) Atrial arrhythmias

      (b) Active peptic ulcer disease

      (c) Gouty arthritis

      (d) Hepatic disease

      (e) Diabetes mellitus

d. **Lovastatin** (Mevacor)

    i. Start at 10 or 20 mg q.d. with evening meal

    ii. Maximum dose: 80 mg q.d.; can give divided doses b.i.d.

        iii. **Warn** about
- (a) Heavy alcohol consumption while on drug
- (b) Risk of myositis (which increases if patient on niacin or gemfibrozil concurrently)
- (c) Possible progression of cataracts

        iv. Monitoring
- (a) Annual eye exam
- (b) SGOT/SGPT before therapy, then at 6 and 12 wk while titrating dose upward, then every 3 mo for first year and periodically thereafter
- (c) CPK should be checked if any symptoms of myositis develop

e. **Pravastatin sodium** (Pravachol)
- i. Starting dose: 10–20 mg q.d.
- ii. Maximum dose: 40 mg q.d.
- iii. **Warn** about risk of myositis and cataracts, as above
- iv. Monitor similarly to lovastatin

2. **For elevated cholesterols and triglycerides**
   a. **Nicotinic acid:** see above for details
   b. **Gemfibrozil** (Lopid)
   - i. Start at 600 mg b.i.d.
   - ii. Take on empty stomach
   - iii. **Warn** of constipation, bloating, and possiblity of gallstones
   - iv. **Avoid** with gallbladder, renal, or hepatic disease
   - v. Use caution in combination with lovastatin because this increases risk of rhabdomyolysis
   - vi. **Monitoring**
     - (a) CBC, SGOT/SGPT, and LDL (for paradoxical rise)
     - (b) Prothrombin time (PT) when patients on warfarin (PT may increase significantly)
     - (c) Glucose in diabetic patient

V. **Monitoring**

A. **All patients** on medical or nonmedical therapy need proper monitoring for
1. Change in cholesterol levels
2. Monitoring adverse effects of drug(s)
3. Support and emphasizing compliance
4. Advice on reducing other cardiovascular risks

B. **For patients on medical therapy**
1. Goals of therapy are as described above in section on phase I diet
2. Repeat nonfasting cholesterol while titrating dosage upward
3. Repeat cholesterol measurements about every 4–6 mo once on stable regimen

4. Consider using combination therapy if single-drug regimen fails to reduce cholesterol to desired levels
   a. Physicians should be wary of drug interactions between cholesterol-lowering medications
C. **Family screening** should be considered
   1. If family history is significant for early CAD or sudden death (<55 y/o)
   2. If familial syndrome is suspected

VI. **Referral to Specialist in Lipid and Cholesterol Disorders for**
   A. Uncertainty of diagnosis or treatment protocols
   B. Patient does not respond to drug therapy
   C. Patient cannot tolerate drugs listed above
   D. Familial syndrome

References

1. Med Lett 30(74), September 9, 1988.
2. National Education Programs Working Group: Report on the Management of Patients with Hypertension and High Blood Cholesterol. Ann Intern Med 114: 224–237, 1991.
3. Report of the National Cholesterol Education Program on Detection, Evaluation, and Treatment of High Blood Cholesterol in Adults. Arch Intern Med 148:36–69, 1988.

Chronic Obstructive Pulmonary Disease

I. **Definition**
   A. Common forms of COPD include emphysema and chronic bronchitis
      1. Emphysema is an alteration in the architecture of the lung characterized by
         a. Irreversible enlargement of the airspaces distal to the terminal bronchiole
         b. Destruction of airspace walls
         c. Absence of pulmonary fibrosis
      2. Chronic bronchitis is characterized by
         a. Chronic progressive cough for >3 mo/yr for 2 or more successive years
         b. Hypertrophy and hyperplasia of mucus glands
         c. Peribronchial fibrosis and mucus plugs

II. **General Principles**
   A. Subgroups of COPD include asthmatic bronchitis and asthma (for details, see chapter on "Asthma")
      1. Asthmatic bronchitis is bronchitis with a bronchospastic component
   B. Most forms of COPD are due to smoking

III. **Diagnostics**

  A. **History**
    1. Symptoms of cough, dyspnea, wheeze
    2. Age at onset
    3. Previous hospitalizations and intubations
    4. Prior and present treatment and medications (including steroids)
    5. Smoking history, including amount, duration, and current use
    6. Environmental/occupational history for inhaled toxins or noxious fumes
    7. Symptoms of right heart failure

  B. **Examination**
    1. Vital signs, respiratory rate
    2. Respiratory evaluation for
       a. Hyperinflation of lungs
       b. Use of accessory muscles for breathing
       c. Abnormal breath sounds
       d. Forced expiration for end-expiratory wheeze
    3. Cardiovascular evaluation
       a. Signs of right heart failure
    4. Clubbing

  C. **Laboratory data**
    1. Investigations, when clinically indicated, may include any of
       a. Spirometric studies and peak flow measurements to indicate
          i. Reduced FEV_1 and peak flow rate
          ii. Reduced FEV_1/FVC ratio
          iii. Reduced DLCO
          iv. Improvement with bronchodilator
       b. Chest x-ray (PA and lateral) for hyperinflation, bullae
       c. Arterial blood gases or oximetry if
          i. Patient has an acute exacerbation
          ii. FEV_1 <1.5 L or EKG indicates right ventricular hypertrophy
          iii. CBC indicates polycythemia
          iv. Patient has severe disease and may benefit from oxygen therapy
          v. It is important to quantify hypercarbia in severe disease
          vi. Oxygen therapy (chronic or short-term) is administered
       d. CBC with indices to detect hypoxia-induced polycythemia
       e. Electrocardiogram to detect
          i. Right ventricular strain
          ii. Atrial arrhythmias
       f. Alpha-1-antiprotease level, which may be useful for evaluating a **young person** with emphysema, especially if there is

      i. No or minimal history of smoking
      ii. No exposure to toxins
      iii. Positive family history for early COPD

IV. **Management**
  A. **General approach**
    1. Smoking cessation should be encouraged in the strongest possible way
    2. Vaccinations
      a. Influenza: yearly for those with COPD/asthma
      b. Pneumococcal: for those >50 y/o with COPD/asthma
    3. Amantadine: when appropriate for those without influenza prophylaxis (see chapter on "Influenza")
    4. When inhalers are prescribed, ensure that patients are instructed on proper use
  B. **Pharmacologic therapy**
    1. **Beta-adrenergic agonists** (usually prescribed as MDIs)
      a. Used in patients with bronchospastic component to disease
        i. Trial of use is beneficial for many patients even if evidence of bronchospasm is not found on clinical examination
      b. Dose as needed up to 2 puffs every 4–6 hr, up to 12 puffs daily
        i. Medium-acting preparations
          (a) Metaproterenol (Alupent)
        ii. Long-acting preparations
          (a) Albuterol (Proventil, Ventolin)
          (b) Terbutaline (Bricanyl)
      c. If difficulty with MDI, try a spacer such as Inspirease
    2. **Corticosteroids** (inhaled or oral)
      a. Acute exacerbations may benefit from short course of oral steroids, especially if
        i. Cough and wheeze have lasted >48 hr without treatment
        ii. Patient has had frequent attacks recently
        iii. Recent attacks have required oral steroids
      b. Usual dose of prednisone is 40 mg q.d. or equivalent
      c. Try to taper off oral steroids within 2 wk
      d. Inhaled steroids useful for helping reduce frequent attacks
        i. Usual dose: 2 puffs q.i.d. (or 3 puffs t.i.d.), up to maximum dosage
          (a) Take after using bronchodilator
        ii. Maximum dosage: 16 puffs daily
        iii. May be started while patient tapers off oral dose
        iv. Rinse mouth and throat after use
      e. Preparations include
        i. Triamcinolone acetonide (Azmacort)
        ii. Beclomethasone dipropionate (Vanceril, Beclovent)

3. **Ipratropium bromide** (Atrovent)
   a. Useful in some patients with COPD
   b. Can try alone or with beta agonists
   c. Usual dose: 2 puffs of MDI aerosol q.i.d.
   d. Maximum dose: 12 puffs/24 hr
4. **Theophylline**
   a. Use is controversial but may help control frequent attacks when bronchodilators and other therapies are inadequate
   b. Monitor level soon after starting drug (e.g., 1 wk)
   c. Initial dose: usually 200–300 mg b.i.d.
   d. Drug preparations are not interchangeable
   e. Serum levels may increase if taken in conjunction with
      i. Cimetidine
      ii. Allopurinol
      iii. Erythromycin
   f. Serum levels may decrease if taken in conjunction with
      i. Cigarette smoking
      ii. Phenytoin
      iii. Rifampin
   g. Toxic symptoms that may occur within therapeutic levels (10–20 μg/ml) include
      i. Nervousness
      ii. Tremor
      iii. GI symptoms
      iv. Arrhythmias and seizures

C. **Oxygen therapy: indication for use is *arterial hypoxemia***
   1. Criteria for O_2 therapy
      a. Patient clinically stable for at least 2 wk
         i. PaO_2 <55 mmHg or O_2 saturation <90% (at rest)
            or
         ii. PaO_2: 55–59 mmHg (at rest) **and** polycythemia or right heart failure/strain
   2. Survival is prolonged if used >18 hr/d but no benefit if used <12–15 hr/d
      a. Preferable use: 24 hr/d
      b. Attempt to raise PaO_2 to 65–80 mmHg or O_2 saturation to 91–95%
         i. In CO_2 retainers raise PaO_2 to 60–70 mmHg range to avoid danger of further CO_2 retention
      c. Start O_2 at low dose (e.g., 1 L by nasal prong)
      d. Monitor PaO_2 or oxygenation as O_2 dose is raised
      e. Increase O_2 by 1 L for sleep and exercise
   3. For patients with nocturnal hypoxemia only
      a. Definition: O_2 saturation <85% while asleep
         i. Sleep study needed to confirm diagnosis
      b. Consider evaluation for nocturnal hypoxemia if PaO_2 >60 mmHg but patient has polycythemia or right ventricular failure
      c. Attempt to increase PaO_2 >60 mmHg at night

4. For patients with exercise hypoxemia
   a. Can measure oxygenation with exercise
   b. No firm consensus on O_2 use in this circumstance
   c. Consult with or refer to pulmonary specialist for advice on O_2 use in this situation

D. **Other therapies**
   1. Breathing exercises may help expectorate sputum
   2. Physical exercise may increase exercise tolerance, but not survival
   3. Chest physical therapy (at home) is useful for patients with cystic fibrosis, bronchiectasis, or chronic bronchitis with >30 cc of sputum production/day

V. **Referral to Specialist for**

A. Uncertainty of diagnosis or treatment
B. Moderate to severe disease with frequent attacks
C. Poor response to simple standard therapies
D. Evaluation and/or monitoring for severe disease
E. Evaluation for oxygen therapy
F. Sleep studies

Reference

American Thoracic Society: Standards for the diagnosis and care of patients with chronic obstructive pulmonary disease (COPD) and asthma. Am Rev Respir Dis 136:225–243, 1987.

Cigarette Smoking

I. **General Principles**

A. Nicotine is about 6 times more addictive than alcohol
B. More than 350,000 persons die yearly because of tobacco-related disease
C. Smoking causes up to $1/3$ of domicile fires in the U.S.
D. Two-thirds of persons who quit do so on their own
E. Many smokers take several tries before finally quitting
F. Physicians must be active in helping people to stop smoking
   1. Giving practical advice and moral support helps
G. Discuss with patients benefits of stopping cigarettes
   1. Increase life expectancy
   2. Increase lung and exercise capacity
   3. Normalize sense of taste and smell
   4. Decrease blood pressure and potential for heart attacks
   5. Stop "smoker's cough"
   6. May improve symptoms of vascular disease
   7. Financial savings from not purchasing cigarettes

II. **Diagnostics**
   A. **History**
      1. Amount smoked per day and when during the day smoking occurs
      2. Duration of smoking habit
      3. Type of cigarette: filter or nonfilter
      4. History of lung diseases
         a. Asthma
         b. Asthmatic bronchitis
         c. Chronic bronchitis
         d. Emphysema
      5. Morning cough
      6. Number of previous attempts at stopping smoking
         a. Duration of successes
         b. Reasons for failure
      7. Symptoms of cardiac and other vascular diseases, including claudication, angina, and cerebrovascular symptoms
      8. Consumption of alcohol (which may increase risk of certain head and neck cancers)
   B. **Examination**
      1. Fingernail clubbing (i.e., lung CA)
      2. Oral examination for precancerous or cancerous lesions
      3. Neck examination for masses/lymph node enlargement
      4. Respiratory exam for signs of COPD or bronchospasm
      5. Signs of right heart failure
   C. **Laboratory data**
      1. Initial investigations are not necessary
      2. For selected patients
         a. See chapter on "COPD" for details
         b. **Note:** chest x-ray for screening for carcinoma is not recommended as a routine test

III. **Management**
   A. **Patients should be given**
      1. Information about benefits of cessation as listed above
      2. Educational materials
      3. Option for smoking cessation program or method
      4. Information about withdrawal
         a. Most symptoms start within 24 hr
         b. Craving for tobacco
            i. Usually worse in the evening and with certain social or environmental cues (e.g., afer dinner or with drinks)
            ii. Subsides in about 1–3 wk
         c. Irritability, anxiety, restlessness are common
         d. Headaches, insomnia, GI upset occur frequently
         e. Appetite often increases, especially for sweets
            i. Average weight gain <10 lbs
            ii. Gain usually **not** permanent

B. **Methods to increase compliance with cessation**
  1. Agree on a quit date and document date in chart
     a. Can have patient sign agreement
  2. Schedule follow-up for 2–3 wk for support
  3. Advise patient to stop cigarettes completely
     a. Tapering can actually prolong withdrawal symptoms
  4. If patient relapses, try again with same or other method
     a. Relapse rate is high
  5. Provide support for cessation at subsequent visits
  6. Advise use of low-calorie snacks and sugar substitutes
  7. Recommend 30 min of exercise, 3–5 times/wk
  8. Ask if patient would like to use nicotine substitute
     a. Nicotine gum (Nicorette)
        i. 1 piece (2 g) chewed over 10 min when craving occurs (gum should not be swallowed)
        ii. Usual dose: 10–12 pieces/d
        iii. Maximum dose: 30 pieces/d
        iv. Taper use after first month
        v. Duration of therapy: usually 3 mo
     b. Nicotine patch (Habitrol, Nicoderm)
        i. Topically q.d.
        ii. Usual duration of therapy: 3 mo
        iii. Avoid using in patients with severe coronary artery disease
        iv. Patient should be made aware of high cost of patch
        v. Patient should **not** wear patch while continuing to smoke

C. **If patient does not want to stop**
  1. State that you, as their physician, advise him/her to stop
  2. Ask what you can say or do to help convince him/her to stop
  3. Document refusal in chart
  4. Repeat sequence of advice and questions next visit

IV. **Referrals for Behavioral Modification**

A. Self-help pamphlets are offered free by
  1. American Lung Association
     a. "Facts About Cigarettes"
     b. "How to Quit Smoking"
     c. National office: (212) 315-8700
     d. Consult telephone directory for local phone numbers
  2. American Cancer Association
     a. "Fresh Start"
     b. National office: (800) 227-2345
     c. Consult telephone directory for local phone numbers
B. Smoking cessation classes include those by
  1. American Lung Association
  2. American Cancer Society
  3. Smokenders: (800) 828-4357
     a. Also offers self-help program

    4. Smoke Watchers
    5. Schick (in Seattle area only): (800) 542-4202
    6. Local hospitals and HMOs
  C. Hypnosis
    1. Of most benefit if patient wants to stop smoking
    2. Hypnosis programs give
      a. Several treatment sessions
      b. Individualized suggestions
      c. Follow-up sessions
  D. Acupuncture
      a. May be helpful for some in suppressing withdrawal symptoms or in supporting other cessation methods

Reference

American College of Physicians: Methods for stopping smoking. Ann Intern Med 105:281–291, 1986.

Colorectal Cancer and Polyps

I. **General Principles**
  A. Incidence of colorectal cancer is about 145,000 cases/yr
  B. It is the second most common cancer in the U.S.
  C. With regard to colorectal polyps
    1. Adenomatous polyps are considered to be precancerous
      a. Prevalence in the U.S. population (>50 y/o) may be up to 30%
      b. About 1% or less develop into cancer
      c. Most polyps are asymptomatic; only a small percent produce detectable GI bleeding
    2. Hyperplastic polyps are not thought to be precancerous
  D. **Persons at increased risk**
    1. Those at high risk
      a. Familial polyposis coli and related disorders
      b. Ulcerative colitis affecting the entire colon
    2. Those at moderate risk
      a. History of previous colonic adenoma or cancer
      b. Left-sided ulcerative colitis
      c. Family history of first-degree relative(s) with colon cancer
      d. Women who have had pelvic radiation for gynecologic malignancy or breast carcinoma
  E. **Persons with average risk** include those in the general population without above risk factors and without clinical evidence of potential colorectal carcinoma (e.g., GI bleeding, abdominal mass, change in bowel habit, abnormal radiologic study)
    1. Patients with clinical evidence of colorectal cancer should not be evaluated by sigmoidoscopy alone

F. **Screening for asymptomatic, average-risk population**
  1. Digital rectal examination after age 40, with fecal occult blood testing (FOBT) yearly after age 50
  2. Flexible sigmoidoscopy every 3–5 yr from age 50
      a. Some screening protocols recommend every year for 2 years, then every 3–5 years thereafter, from age 50
  3. Hemoccult testing has relatively poor sensitivity and specificity
      a. False negative and positive rates as high as 30%
      b. In order to optimize results of hemoccult testing
          i. Avoid extended storage of specimens as this may cause false negatives
          ii. Advise patient on foods to be avoided within 48 hr of hemoccult testing
              (a) No vitamin C or iron-containing compounds (including vitamins) or NSAIDs/aspirin
              (b) Avoid red meats and vegetables with high peroxidase activity such as broccoli, turnips, cauliflower, and radishes

II. **Diagnostics**

   A. **History**
     1. Persistent change in bowel habit
         a. Constipation, diarrhea, or tenesmus
     2. History of inflammatory bowel disease
     3. Presence of abdominal pain, often cramping in nature
     4. Rectal bleeding of any type
     5. History of recent microcytic, hypochromic, or iron-deficiency anemia
     6. Medications: NSAIDs and aspirin-containing preparations
     7. Family history: polyposis, GI tract cancers

   B. **Examination**
     1. Abdominal palpation for
         a. Hepatic enlargement
         b. Masses
     2. Rectal examination yearly after age 40 for rectal masses
     3. Hemoccult test after age 50

   C. **Laboratory data**
     1. **Routine screening for average-risk asymptomatic patients**
         a. Flexible sigmoidoscopy (35-mm or 60-mm endoscope) every 3–5 yr
     2. **Further investigations for properly administered *positive* hemoccult test**
         a. Refer for colonoscopy **or**
         b. Sigmoidoscopy plus double-contrast barium enema
         c. **Note:** patients with a positive hemoccult test should also be considered for upper GI evaluation, especially if there are upper GI symptoms or lower GI assessment is nondiagnostic

      d. If a polyp is found on sigmoidoscopy, refer for colonoscopy and polypectomy(ies)

      e. **If the barium study indicates a possible polyp** or lesion, refer for colonoscopy

  3. **In patients with ulcerative colitis**

      a. For universal colitis after 8–10 yr

         i. Colonoscopy yearly, with multiple biopsies

      b. For left-sided colitis after 15–20 yr

         i. Colonoscopy every 1–2 yr, with biopsies

  4. **In patients with a previous adenoma or carcinoma in situ**

      a. Colonoscopy 1 yr after initial study

         i. If patient is polyp-free at that time, advise colonoscopy every 3–5 yr

         ii. If polyp was large, sessile benign adenoma, then follow-up colonoscopy is done within 6 mo to ensure polyp's complete excision

  5. **For patients after surgical resection for colorectal cancer**

      a. For first 5 yr after surgery, periodic evaluations include

         i. Clinical evaluation and FOBT

         ii. LFTs and CEA

         iii. Sigmoidoscopy or colonoscopy, depending on site of lesion

         iv. Chest x-rays

      b. Intervals for monitoring in the first 5 yr should be discussed with GI specialist

      c. After 5 yr, with no indication of disease, evaluations include

         i. Clinical evaluation and FOBT yearly

         ii. Colonoscopy every 3 yr

III. **Referral to Gastroenterologist or Other Endoscopic Specialist for**

  A. Abnormal barium study indicating possible polyp or cancer or other potentially dangerous lesion

  B. Presence of a polyp on sigmoidoscopy

  C. A persistent positive FOBT with nondiagnostic sigmoidoscopy and double-contrast barium enema

  D. Monitoring after surgical resection of cancer

  E. Colonoscopy

References

1. American Gastroenterological Association, American Society for Gastrointestinal Endoscopy: Detection and surveillance of colorectal cancer. JAMA 261:580–585, 1989.
2. American Cancer Society: Guidelines for the Cancer-related Checkup. American Cancer Society, 1991.

D

Dementia

I. **Definition**

  A. **Dementia is characterized** by
1. **Absence of fluctuating mental state** (delirium)
2. Impaired memory
3. Impaired abstraction, judgment, or higher cortical function
4. Personality changes
5. Impaired function in social and/or occupational activities
6. Absence of other organic causes

II. **General Principles**

  A. **Delirium** can infrequently be chronic and may closely mimic the often insidious onset of dementia

  B. Be wary of **drugs** causing low-grade delirium

  C. **Depression** may mimic or exacerbate dementia

  D. Cognitive impairment is often subtle in initial stages and may be difficult to differentiate from a patient's usual status

III. **Diagnostics**

  A. **History**
1. Duration and progression of cognitive impairment(s)
2. Stability of mental state (e.g., fluctuating)
3. Medications and alcohol
4. Cardiovascular history (CHD, TIAs, CVAs)
5. Systemic symptoms of thyroid disease, carcinoma
6. History of syphilis, anemia

  B. **Examination**
1. General mental state for alertness, orientation
2. Neck examination for thyroid enlargement
3. Neurologic examination, including positional and vibration senses, reflexes (B_{12} deficiency)
4. Thorough physical examination searching for potentially reversible forms of dementia

  C. **Screening in selected persons**
1. The Folstein Mini-Mental State Exam (MMSE) (see Appendix 5, p. 288) is a 5–10-min screening tool
   - a. A total of 30 points is possible; scores of less than 24 indicate increased probability of cognitive impairment
   - b. Serial MMSEs may also be useful for following patients' cognitive changes
   - c. Low scores may occur with delirium
   - d. Persons with little or no education score poorly

    e. Race and gender are not associated with poor results

    f. A small percent of people score low for no identifiable reason

D. Laboratory data

1. **Routine** (with abbreviated list of reasons for ordering)

    a. CBC and differential (anemia may worsen cognitive function)

    b. ESR (considered significant if significantly elevated, suggestive of vasculitis, malignancy, or chronic infection)

    c. Serum VDRL test

    d. Thyroid function tests (TSH and FTI)

    e. Urinalysis (renal dysfunction, chronic infection)

    f. Chest x-ray (for malignancy or severe lung disease)

    g. Electrolytes, urea, and creatinine (renal failure, hyponatremia)

    h. Metabolites: Ca, Mg, P

    i. LFTs (hepatic dysfunction as a possible cause of dementia)

    j. Serum B_{12} and rbc folate (deficiencies may present as dementia)

    k. EKG (bradycardias or low cardiac ouptut may present as cognitive dysfunction)

2. **Further investigations** may include any of

    a. Depression screening

        i. Clinicians should have a high index of suspicion for depression because it is often missed and can mimic or exacerbate cognitive impairment

    b. Neuropsychological testing can help with

        i. Early dementia in person of high intelligence

        ii. Obtaining baseline to monitor changes in possible dementia

        iii. Differentiating from depression and delirium

        iv. Obtaining information on impairment of specific cerebral function

    c. LP, if neurosyphilis or other infection suspected

    d. CT scan if history or physical exam suggests

        i. A mass lesion

        ii. Previous CVA(s)

        iii. Normal pressure hydrocephalus dementia

        iv. Dementia is of brief duration (e.g., <1 yr) and/or rapidly progressive

    e. EEG, if altered consciousness or possibility of seizures

    f. MRI scan in place of CT scan may pick up smaller lesions but is considerably more expensive

    g. HIV test should be considered in persons who are young or who have other signs or HIV disease or who have known risk factors for HIV infection

IV. **Management**

  A. **General approach**

    1. Address other medical conditions

    2. Ensure that there is adequate care for patient at home (Meals on Wheels, nursing aides, home help, as needed)

    3. Ask if there is adequate support for caregivers

    4. Discuss with family the prognosis and natural history of progressive cognitive impairment (Note: survival may be 2–20 yr, averaging about 7 yr)

  B. **Helpful measures** may include

    1. Avoiding **drugs with anticholinergic effects** (these may worsen dementia)

    2. Avoiding polypharmacy

    3. Referral to **day-care centers** to help patient socialization and to give a respite to family members

    4. Referral to **occupational therapy** for orientation therapies and for help in ensuring home safety

    5. Referral to **social worker**

    6. Group therapy and family counseling

  C. **Recommend**

    1. Family should clarify **patient's wishes** (regarding future care and extraordinary measures) while patient is still cognizant

    2. **Financial and legal arrangements** (durable power of attorney, durable power for health care) be made

    3. Family contact the Alzheimer's Association and/or other local **support groups**

V. **Referral to Geriatric Care Team or Specialist for**

  A. Uncertainty of diagnosis or management

  B. Assistance with care plan or with helping family cope

  C. Follow-up care and monitoring of physical and/or mental function

  D. Assistance in functional assessment

References

1. National Institutes of Health: Differential diagnosis of dementing diseases. JAMA 259:3411–3416, 1987.
2. Siu AL: Screening for dementia and investigating its causes. Ann Intern Med 115:122–132, 1991.

Depression

I. **Definition**

  A. Depression is a catchphrase for distinct categories of dysphoria often **classified as**

1. Affective disorders, including major depression
   a. Melancholia (endogenous depression)
   b. Psychotic depression
2. Organic mood disorder (secondary to medical illness)
3. Adjustment disorder (grief reaction, life changes)
4. Dysthymia (prolonged low-grade depressive symptoms)

B. Depression may be a presenting symptom for other psychiatric disorders (e.g., schizoaffective disease or anxiety state)

II. General Principles

A. It is important to recognize and act on symptoms of depression
B. Incidence of major depression is about 6–10% in primary care patients
C. Depression often has a self-limiting course of 6 mo to 2 yr
D. Depression in elderly can present as progressive dementia
E. **Drugs that may precipitate or worsen depressive state**
   1. Alcohol (or any substance abuse)
   2. Antihypertensives: beta blockers, clonidine, methyldopa
   3. Benzodiazepines and sedatives
   4. Cimetidine
   5. Narcotic analgesics
   6. Steroids
F. **Criteria for major depression and related disorders** (DSM-III-R)
   1. Major depression
      a. Dysphoria **or** loss of pleasure/interest in usual activities
      b. At least 4 of the following present **nearly every day** for at least 2 wk
         i. Appetite/weight: significant loss or gain
         ii. Sleep disturbances: insomnia or hypersomnia
         iii. Psychomotor changes: agitation or retardation
         iv. Anhedonia
         v. Fatigue or loss of energy
         vi. Guilt or feelings of worthlessness/hopelessness
         vii. Inability to concentrate/think clearly
         viii. Suicidal/death ideation
      c. Neither of the following should predominate presentation
         i. Bizarre behavior
         ii. Obsession with hallucinations or delusions without congruent change in mood
      d. Not associated with schizophrenic, schizophreniform, or paranoid disorder
      e. Not due to organic cause or bereavement
   2. Once major depression is diagnosed, then **melancholic (endogenous)** depression is defined by 5 or more of
      a. Loss of pleasure or interest in usual activities
      b. Lack of excitement for previously stimulating activities
      c. Worse symptoms in morning

      d. Report from observer of psychomotor retardation/agitation

      e. Marked loss of weight or appetite

      f. Previous depressive episode(s), followed by partial or complete recovery(ies)

      g. Lack of personality change before first depressive episode

      h. Good response to therapy in prior depressive episode(s)

      i. Early morning awakening

  3. **Dysthymia** is characterized by

      a. Depressed mood for >2 yr

      b. Two or more symptoms listed in category b (above) for major depression on a daily or near daily basis

III. Diagnostics

  A. **History** (see also criteria below)

    1. General mood

    2. Duration of symptoms

    3. Recent life experiences

    4. Alcohol and substance abuse

    5. Medications

    6. Family history of alcohol abuse, suicide, depression, or manic-depression

    7. Previous psychiatric diagnoses/treatments

    8. Previous episodes of depressive symptoms

    9. Manic symptoms

      a. Hyperactivity >2 wk

      b. Binges: e.g., buying, creative activity, or drinking

      c. Rapidity of speech or actions

    10. Preoccupations with guilt, disease, or hopelessness

    11. Suicidal ideation or suicide attempts

    12. Review for systemic disease(s)

  B. **Examination**

    1. General mental and physical state

    2. Scars from previous suicide attempts or episodes of self-harm

    3. Signs of thyroid or other endocrine disease

    4. Signs of systemic disorder

    5. Neurologic examination

    6. **Mental status examination includes**

      a. General appearance: mode and tidiness of dress

      b. Orientation and level of consciousness

      c. Affect and mood

      d. Attention span

      e. Speech: fluency, coherence, tangential thoughts

      f. Obsessional speech or behavior(s)

      g. Psychotic behavior: delusions or hallucinations

      h. Cognitive ability

      i. Judgment and insight

      j. Suicidal ideation or intent

C. **Laboratory data**
   1. **Initial investigation**
      a. Thyroid function: TSH and FT4 or FTI
   2. **If diagnosis is uncertain, organic disease suspected, or with severe depression,** or if patient is elderly, consider
      a. ESR
      b. CBC
      c. Electrolytes, Cr, BUN
      d. Metabolites, Ca, P, Mg
      e. Liver function tests

IV. **Management**

A. **General approach**
   1. **Symptoms,** not exact diagnoses, are used for determining treatment
      a. For **delusional, psychotic** patients, refer immediately to psychiatric care
      b. For **nondelusional, severely depressed** patients (catatonic, suicidal/homicidal), refer for further management to psychiatric facility
      c. For **nondelusional but melancholic depression** (without above features)
         i. Drug therapy **and** psychotherapy are often combined for maximal treatment
         ii. Psychotherapy may be administered by
            (a) Psychologist or therapist
            (b) Pyschiatric outpatient
      d. For **nondelusional, uncomplicated** depression (e.g., dysthymia)
         i. Psychotherapy/psychiatric or primary physician counseling may be of great benefit and may alleviate need for medication
         ii. Trial of medication if depressive symptoms persist
   2. **Monitoring**
      a. Follow patient closely (once per 1–2 wk) for at least 6–8 wk
      b. Counsel family on disorder, treatment, and prognosis
      c. Advise patient to refrain from major life changes until depression has resolved

B. **Pharmacologic therapy**
   1. **General principles**
      a. It is helpful to become familiar with profile of several drugs (from the different categories)
      b. Antidepressants are most helpful when there are specific target symptoms such as insomnia, loss of appetite, decreased concentration, or other vegetative signs
      c. For proper trial of medication, use maintenance dose and give duration of >4–6 wk before declaring trial a failure

    d. Tricyclics (Table 1) are generally considered first-line drugs

       i. Dosing considerations

         (a) Usually can raise dose about every 3–5 d

         (b) Reduce dose by about 50% in elderly and infirm

      ii. Side effects include (consult drug manual for specifics)

         (a) Sedation (more with amitriptyline, doxepin)

         (b) Anticholinergic (less with desipramine, nortriptyline)

         (c) Orthostasis (less with despiramine, nortriptyline, and protriptyline)

      iii. Contraindications include

         (a) Conduction defects (including blocks or worsening conduction defects after starting)

         (b) Unstable cardiac disease (including acute period after MI)

         (c) Uncontrolled glaucoma

      iv. Special considerations

         (a) Limit quantity (1–2 wk) to avoid dangerous overdose

         (b) Usually give q.h.s. because of drowsiness in initial stages

         (c) Sedative effects are often useful for sleeplessness

         (d) Orthostatic effects may be pronounced in elderly

         (e) Clomipramine is helpful with obsessive-compulsive behaviors

         (f) Imipramine and desipramine are helpful with panic/anxiety states

    e. Treatment (for responders) should last 6–12 mo

    f. When discontinuing medication, taper over 1 wk to avoid withdrawal symptoms

TABLE 1. Tricyclics (Selected Listing) by Drug, Dose, Incremental Increase, Usual Maintenance Dose, and Monitoring

Drug	Dose (mg q.h.s.)			Plasma Levels (ng/ml)
	Initial	Raise by	Maintenance (Maximum)	
Amitriptyline	25–75	25	150 (300)	Not routine
Clomipramine	25	25	100 (250)	Not routine
Desipramine	25–75	25	200 (300)	Not routine
Doxepin	25–75	25	150 (300)	Not routine
Imipramine	25–75	25	150 (300)	Not routine
Nortriptyline	25–50	25	100 (150)	50–150
Protriptyline	5–15	5–10	40 (60)	70–170

TABLE 2. Newer Agents (Selected Listing) by Drug, Dose, Incremental Increase, Usual Maintenance Dose, and Monitoring

Drug	Dose (mg)			
	Initial	Raise by	Maintenance	Monitor
			(Maximum)	
Fluoxetine	20 q.a.m.	20	20–80 q.a.m. (80)	Not routine
Trazodone	50 t.i.d.	50	50–100 t.i.d. (400/d)	Not routine
Maprotiline	25 q.d.	25	25–150 q.d. (200)	Not routine

    g. After drug is discontinued, see patient within 1 mo for reassessment and symptoms/signs of relapse

    h. Newer drugs (Table 2) may also be considered

       i. Dosing considerations

         (a) If needed, increase fluoxetine after about 2 wk

           (i) Others can be raised every 3–5 d

         (b) For fluoxetine: doses above 20 q.a.m. go to b.i.d. schedule

         (c) Use lower doses in elderly and infirm

       ii. Adverse effects

         (a) Fluoxetine: hyperactivity, insomnia, mania, anorexia

         (b) Trazodone: priapism, sedation

         (c) Maprotiline: anticholinergic effects

       iii. Special considerations

         (a) Sedative effect of trazodone may help with agitation, sleeplessness

         (b) Fluoxetine should be used with caution if patient is diabetic because it may alter blood glucose

    i. **Monoamine oxidase inhibitors** (MAOI) are often used as alternatives to tricyclic therapy

         (a) Consult psychiatrist for dosage and protocols

         (b) Ensure patient has received warnings on contraindicated drugs and foods/substances to be avoided while on MAOIs

V. **Referral to Psychiatrist and/or Psychologist for**

    A. Uncertainty of diagnosis or management

    B. Failure to improve within 1 mo

    C. Worsening of depression while receiving treatment

    D. Noncompliance with medical treatment

    E. Recurrent symptoms after treatment

    F. Detoxification for substance abuse

    G. Melancholic or severe depression

    H. When depression is a manifestation of other psychiatric disorder

References

1. Goldberg RJ: Depression in primary care: DSM-III diagnoses and other depressive syndromes. J Gen Intern Med 3:492–497, 1988.
2. McGreevey JF, Franco K: Depression in the elderly: The role of the primary care physician in management. J Gen Intern Med 3:498–507, 1988.
3. Potter WZ, Rudorfer MV, Manji H: The pharmacologic treatment of depression. N Engl J Med 325:633–642, 1991.

Diabetes Mellitus

I. **Definition**

  A. This heterogeneous syndrome manifested by hyperglycemia may be classified as follows

    1. **Diabetes mellitus** (DM)

      a. **DM type I**

        i. Insulin-dependent type (IDDM)

        ii. Insulin deficient due to islet cell loss

        iii. Ketosis prone

        iv. Occurs at any age, common in youth

      b. **DM type II**

        i. Non–insulin-dependent type (NIDDM)

          (a) Patients, however, may require insulin for good glucose control

        ii. Ketosis resistant

        iii. Majority are overweight adults

      c. **Diabetes associated with certain conditions**

        i. Pancreatic disease, drug- or chemical-induced

        ii. Endocrinopathies, genetic syndromes

      d. **Criteria for diagnosis in DM**

        i. Plasma glucose >200 mg/dl with symptoms

        ii. Fasting plasma glucose (FPG) ≥140 mg/dl on 2 occasions

        iii. FPG <140 mg/dl but >115 mg/dl and 2 oral glucose tolerance tests (OGTTs) with 75 g glucose load resulting in

          (a) Plasma glucose of ≥200 mg/dl after 2 hr

          (b) One or more intervening plasma glucoses >200 mg/dl

    2. **Gestational diabetes**

      a. **Criteria for diagnosis in gestational diabetes**

        i. Two or more of the following with a 100-g glucose load

          (a) FPG >105 mg/dl

          (b) 1 hr >190 mg/dl

          (c) 2 hr >165 mg/dl

          (d) 3 hr >145 mg/dl

3. **Impaired glucose tolerance** (IGT)
   a. Intermediate between normal and overt diabetes
   b. **Criteria for diagnosis of IGT**
      i. FPG <140 but >115 mg/dl
      ii. 2-hr postprandial glucose ≥140 and <200 mg/dl
      iii. 1 intervening value of ≥200 mg/dl after a 75-g oral glucose load

II. **Diagnostics**

A. **History**
1. Polydipsia, polyuria, polyphagia, weight loss
2. Weight history and nutritional status
3. Exercise history
4. History of prior infections (dental, foot, GU, skin)
5. History of diabetic complications, including kidney disease, sexual dysfunction, peripheral vascular disease, fluctuating changes in vision, vaginal discharge and pruritus (candidiasis), or other fungal infections such as tinea pedis or cruris
6. Family history of diabetes
7. Psychosocial issues that might influence the management of diabetes

B. **Examination**
1. Height and weight
2. Blood pressure
3. Ophthalmoscopic examination
4. Dental and periodontal
5. Thyroid palpation
6. Cardiac examination
7. Pulses (looking for bruits and diminished pulses)
8. Foot examination (looking between toes)
9. Neurological (sensory, motor, myopathy)
10. Also, look for signs of secondary causes of diabetes
    a. Hemochromatosis (skin pigmentation)
    b. Pancreatic disease
    c. Acromegaly, Cushing's syndrome

C. **Laboratory data**
1. Usual investigations in a diabetic include
   a. Fasting plasma glucose
   b. Glycosylated hemoglobin
   c. Fasting lipid profile (cholesterol, triglycerides, LDL, HDL)
   d. Serum electrolytes, creatinine, and BUN
   e. Urinalysis (proteinuria, ketones)
2. Further investigations may include any of
   a. Thyroid function test (especially in type 1 DM): TSH, and FT4 or FTI
   b. Electrocardiogram, especially for older diabetics
   c. Electrolytes and anion gap should be considered if serum glucose >350 mg/dl and/or urine testing indicates significant ketones

i. If anion gap is noted, check serum pH or ABGs for acidosis

d. Oral glucose tolerance test is sometimes done when diagnosis suspected but tests are nondiagnostic (e.g., FBS >115 mg/dl but <140 mg/dl)

III. **Management**

A. **Patient education**

1. Patients on hypoglycemic agents should always carry sugar or glucose tablet (available in stores) or equivalent (i.e., candy bar)
2. The patient should understand
   a. Goals (desired blood glucose level)
   b. Medications and possible side effects
   c. Nutrition recommendations
      i. Initial referral to a dietician is a must to individualize goals
      ii. Sodium intake not to exceed 3 g/d
      iii. Moderate alcohol (2 or fewer drinks/d)
      iv. Alternative sweeteners such as aspartame (Nutrasweet)
      v. Routine timing of meals and snacks
      vi. Weight management in the overweight
      vii. Cooking and diet instruction to patient and/or to the cook in the family
   d. Diabetic care regimens such as
      i. Foot hygiene and observation for blisters or other skin changes (see below)
      ii. Periodic eye examinations (see below)
      iii. Recognition of hypoglycemic symptoms
   e. Causes and symptoms of ketosis (see below)
3. **Lifestyle changes**
   a. Cessation of smoking and moderation of alcohol intake
4. **Exercise**
   a. Care should be given to those with risk factors for CAD
      i. Consider an ETT for those older than 35 yr, especially if there are any clinical signs of CAD
   b. Advise aerobic exercise at 50–70% max capacity for 20–60 min, 3–5 times/wk
   c. Warmups and cool downs
   d. Avoid extreme heat or cold
   e. Proper footwear used and feet inspected daily after exercise
   f. Hydration should be maintained
   g. Blood glucose monitored before, during, and after exercise
   h. Patients should carry sugar or similar in case of hypoglycemia during exercise
5. **Self-monitoring of blood and/or urine glucose**

     a. Use of a record system (daily or q.o.d.) once patient on stable regimen of hypoglycemic medications

     b. Of preferable use is blood glucose, but some patients will not comply with this

6. **Symptoms and treatment of hypoglycemia**

     a. Symptoms include anxiousness, palpitations, sweating, behavioral changes, faintness, lightheadedness, hunger, headache, trembling, and nightmares

     b. Treatment may include use of candy, sweets, juice, or anything with sugar in it

        i. Some patients use glucagon, 1-mg injections, IM or SQ

     c. Family members should understand symptoms and treatment of hypoglycemia

7. **For patients who are ketosis prone**

     a. Wear a bracelet or necklace that states patient's diagnosis of diabetes

     b. Discuss how to prevent DKA

     c. Discuss symptoms of DKA: nausea, vomiting, altered mental status

8. **For the diabetic female of childbearing age**

     a. Provide information on risks involved if she becomes pregnant

        i. Risks of birth defects

        ii. Need for prepregnancy care

9. **Potential complications of diabetes with awareness of preventive measures in**

     a. Vision

     b. Cardiovascular disease

     c. Renal dysfunction

     d. Foot ulcers and infections (see below)

     e. Neurological impairment

     f. Vascular disease and impotence

10. **Preventive measures for periodontal disease**

     a. Brushing teeth with soft tooth brush twice a day

     b. Preventive dental care every 6 months

     c. Scheduling dental appointments that do not interfere with insulin or meal schedule

B. **Special considerations: hypertension in the diabetic**

     1. Higher incidence in the socioeconomically disadvantaged

     2. Contributes substantially to morbidity and mortality in association with diabetes

     a. Even moderate elevated pressure may increase incidence of renal dysfunction

     3. Nonpharmacologic attempts to reduce BP include

     a. Diet and exercise

     b. Low-sodium intake

     c. Moderate alcohol of <2 drinks/d

     d. See chapter on "Hypertension" for details and on when to begin drug therapy, if necessary

4. Attempt to avoid drugs that induce or worsen autonomic neuropathy or complications of diabetes such as
     a. Hypoglycemia awareness masked by beta blockers
     b. Orthostatic hypotension with thiazides and other diuretics
     c. Impotence with beta blockers (as well as other antihypertensives)
     d. Lipid profile may be worsened by
          i. Beta blockers, thiazides

5. ACE inhibitors and calcium channel blockers are often good choices
     a. ACE inhibitors may decrease diabetic proteinuria, but care must be taken in those with renal dysfunction

C. **Pharmacologic therapy of diabetes**
  1. **Initiating therapy for non-insulin-dependent diabetic**
     a. For moderate blood sugar elevation, consider
          i. Diet control
               and
          ii. Exercising regularly
     b. If these fail to control blood sugar, consider an oral hypoglycemic agent
          i. **Sulfonylureas**
            (a) Stimulate the secretion of insulin from the pancreas and increase the number of insulin receptors
            (b) Contraindicated in
               (i) Pregnant women
               (ii) Those allergic to sulfa drugs
            (c) Use cautiously with thiazides, barbiturates, warfarin, and aspirin
            (d) **Second-generation agents** are the most commonly used oral hypoglycemics
               (i) **Glyburide** (DiaBeta, Micronase)
                  • Duration: 24 hr; t ½ =10 hr
                  • Can be started at 2.5 mg/d
                  • Maximum dose is 20 mg/d
               (ii) **Glipizide** (Glucotrol)
                  • Duration: 10–24 hr; t ½ = 2–4 hr
                  • Usually started at 5 mg b.i.d.
                  • Maximum dose is 20 mg b.i.d.
                  • Glipizide should be taken at least 30 min prior to a meal
            (e) **First-generation agents**
               (i) **Chlorpropamide** (Diabinese)
                  • Duration: 1–3 d; t ½ = 36 hr
                  • Daily dose: 100–750 mg in single dose
                  • Excreted unchanged by kidneys

- Contraindicated in patients with chronic renal failure
- Disulfiram-like reaction may occur with alcohol

  (ii) **Tolbutamide** (Orinase)
- Duration: 6–12 hr; t ½ = 4–5 hr
- Can be given in divided doses from 500 mg to 3.0 g/d

  (iii) **Tolazamide** (Tolinase)
- Duration: 12–24 hr; t ½ = 7 hr
- Can be given in single or divided dose from 0.1–1.0 g

2. **Insulin therapy**
   a. Should be given when patient
      i. Becomes ketotic without insulin therapy
      ii. When diet, exercise, and oral hypoglycemic agents fail to control blood sugar adequately
         - This use may need to be only temporary if blood sugar control improves with weight loss, diet control, and/or exercise
   b. Duration and onset of action depend on brand and type of insulin
   c. **Types of insulin**
      i. **Regular** (short-acting)
         (a) Onset of action: .5–1 hr
         (b) Peak action: 2–3 hr
         (c) Duration: 5–7 hr
      ii. **Semilente**
         (a) Onset of action: .5–3 hr
         (b) Peak action: 4–7 hr
         (c) Duration: 12–16 hr
      iii. **Lente** (intermediate-acting)
         (a) Onset: 1–2.5 hr
         (b) Peak action: 7–15 hr
         (c) Duration: 18–24 hr
      iv. **NPH** (intermediate-acting)
         (a) Onset of action: 1–2 hr
         (b) Peak action: 4–12 hr
         (c) Duration: 18–24 hr
      v. **Ultralente** (long-acting)
         (a) Onset of action: 4–6 hr
         (b) Peak action: 16–18 hr
         (c) Duration: 36 hr
   d. **Adverse reactions to insulin**
      i. Rare to have systemic allergic reaction
      ii. Most reactions are local reactions that commonly begin in first weeks after initiating therapy
      iii. Reactions are often seen in less pure preparations
   e. **Initiating insulin therapy**

    i. Insulin can be used in a variety of ways and regimens and to some degree is based on trials of use as well as motivation of patient

      (a) Some commonly used methods include

        (i) NPH only in the morning, 30–60 min before breakfast

        (ii) A split regimen with NPH/Regular in the morning and NPH/Regular in the evening if necessary
- See below for details

        (iii) Continuous pump
- For motivated patients only

        (iv) In combination with oral hypoglycemic agent
- Efficacy is controversial and may only increase costs
- Patients may benefit from such therapy if total insulin dose >100 U/d

    ii. **To estimate initial insulin doses**

      (a) Calculate total daily insulin requirements

        (i) If not exposed to exogenous insulin, start at 0.4–0.6 U/kg of lean body weight

        (ii) If obese, insulin resistance is possible; start at 0.6 U/kg of lean body weight

    iii. **Timing of administration**

      (a) If single daily dose is not optimal, consider a split-and-mixed regimen, for instance

        (i) $2/3$ of total insulin given in a.m.
- $2/3$ NPH
- $1/3$ Regular

        (ii) $1/3$ of total insulin given in p.m.
- ½ NPH
- ½ Regular

    iv. **A numerical example of the above**

      (a) In a 60-kg person, the estimated daily dose is 30 U of insulin, which may be given as

        (i) 30 U NPH in a.m.
            or

        (ii) 20 U NPH/10 U Regular in a.m.
            or

        (iii) 13 U NPH/7 U Regular in a.m. and 5 U NPH/5 U Regular in p.m.

3. **Continuing care and ambulatory monitoring**

  a. Frequency of follow-up visits depends on difficulty of obtaining glucose control

  b. Once stable, patients should be seen every 3–6 mo

    i. Review record of glucose monitoring

    ii. Reassess patient knowledge of diabetes and self-management skills annually

      iii. Physical exam at least annually
         (a) Monitor weight and BP
         (b) Fundal examination
      iv. Examine feet carefully
         (a) Toenail care
         (b) Fissuring between toes
         (c) Superficial ulcers and blistering
         (d) Pulses
         (e) Sensory examination
      v. If sensorimotor deficits are noted, consider
         (a) Footwear modifications
         (b) Toenail management and footcare by podiatrist
      vi. **Laboratory data for monitoring**
         (a) Glycosylated hemoglobin and FBG at least semiannually
         (b) Lipid profile and creatinine/BUN annually
         (c) LFTs every 6–12 mo if patient on oral hypoglycemics
         (d) Urinalysis yearly with 24-hr urine protein determination if significant protein found on urinalysis
            (i) Microalbuminuria method preferred when available

4. **Eye care**
  a. For patients with type I diabetes (IDDM), annual screening begins 5 yr after the onset of diabetes
  b. Patients with type II diabetes need baseline examination after diagnosis
    i. If normal examination by dilated ophthalmoscopy, reassess annually
    ii. If normal examination by 7-field stereoscopic photographs, reassess after 4 yr, followed by annual eye evaluation
  c. Promptly refer patients with abnormal fundoscopic examination to an ophthalmologist

5. **Foot care**
  a. Patient should have instructions on
    i. Foot hygiene and inspection of feet daily for cuts and breaks in skin
    ii. Wearing properly fitted and supportive footwear and breaking in new shoes slowly
    iii. Cutting toenails straight across
    iv. Avoid foot trauma and walking barefoot
    v. Seeking care for
       (a) A foot infection of any type
       (b) A foot ulcer
       (c) A non-healing blister
       (d) Areas of persistent redness or irritation

6. **Hospital admission guidelines**

   a. Ketoacidosis (pH <7.35) and serum bicarbonate <15
      mEq/L and ketonemia or ketonuria
      i. DKA can occur at any serum glucose level
   b. Poor control requiring close monitoring
   c. New-onset diabetics with very high blood glucose
   d. Hyperosmolar state with impaired mental status
      i. For calculation of osmolar gap, see "Useful Equa-
         tions" (Appendix 6, p. 289)
   e. Recurrent or persistent hypoglycemia (especially if
      caused by sulfonylurea)
   f. Institution of insulin-pump therapy

IV. **Referral to an Endocrinologist and/or Diabetic Clinic for**
   A. Uncertainty of diagnosis or management
   B. Education on diet, exercise, or other components of diabetic
      management
   C. Monitoring of fragile or difficult to control diabetics
   D. Gestational diabetes

References

1. American Diabetes Association: Clinical practice recommendations, 1980–
   1990. Diabetes Care 14(Suppl 2), 1991.
2. The Prevention and Treatment of Complications of Diabetes Mellitus: A
   Guide for Primary Care Practitioners. Department of Health and Human
   Services, Centers for Disease Control, National Center for Chronic Disease
   Prevention and Health Promotion, Atlanta, 1991.
3. American College of Physicians, American Diabetes Association, and American Academy of Ophthalmology: Screening guidelines for diabetic retinopathy. Ann Intern Med 116:683–685, 1992.
4. Working Group on Hypertension in Diabetes: Statement on hypertension in
   diabetes mellitus. Final report. Arch Intern Med 147:830–843, 1987.

E

Eating Disorders: Anorexia Nervosa and Bulimia

I. Definition

A general definition is ritualized activities to lose or control weight by abnormal eating behaviors, purging, and/or excessive exercise

II. Criteria (DSM-III-R)

A. **Anorexia nervosa**
   1. Intense fear of gaining weight even when underweight or emaciated
   2. Refusal to maintain even minimal normal body weight: weight loss of $>15\%$ from original or projected body weight by height and weight chart (if <18 y/o)
   3. Distorted perception of body image
   4. Amenorrhea: absence without apparent cause of at least three consecutive menses
   5. No organic cause found to explain weight reduction

B. **Bulimia nervosa**
   1. Recurrent binges (usually of high caloric foods): averaging at least 2/wk for 3 or more mo
   2. Feeling unable to control urge to eat during binges
   3. Regular use of self-induced vomiting, laxatives, diuretics, strict dieting, or exercise to stop weight gain
   4. Persistent worry about body image
   5. Other characteristics include
      a. Inconspicuous, rapid consumption of foods
      b. Ending a binge by sleep, abdominal pain, or vomiting
      c. Post-binge depression/anguish

III. General Principles

A. About 10% of patients have symptoms of bulimia and anorexia
B. Prevalence in adolescents and young women is estimated 10–15%
   1. Bulimia may affect up to 20% of college women
   2. Other groups susceptible to bulimia
      a. Jockeys
      b. Ballet dancers and models
      c. Gymnasts
      d. Wrestlers
      e. Actors and actresses
C. Both disorders occur primarily in females (90% of cases)

D. Bulimics often appear healthy, but an estimated 90% may have depressive symptoms or suffer from clinical depression

E. Mortality approaches 6% in anorexics, mostly from starvation or suicide

IV. Diagnostics

A. History includes questions about
1. Repeated attempts at dieting and with trying new diets
2. Weight fluctuations and/or weight loss
3. Binging on foods, frequency of binges, postbinge depression
4. Use of laxatives and diuretics
5. Eating when anxious, upset, or depressed
6. Use of over-exercise or starvation to control weight
7. Secondary amenorrhea (from loss >17% of original weight)
8. Binging when alone but not when other people are around
9. Family dynamics and alcohol use

B. Examination
1. General physical appearance
2. General mental and cognitive status
3. Teeth (stains and decay from vomiting)
4. Evaluation of sexual and breast development
5. Type of hair on body
   a. Lanugo hair often seen in anorexics

C. Laboratory data
1. For selected patients, depending on presentation
   a. CBC and differential
      i. Anoretics may develop anemia, leukopenia, thrombocytopenia
   b. Electrolytes, Cr, BUN (can get severe hypokalemia with vomiting)
   c. LFTs, albumin, and total protein
   d. Metabolites: Ca, P, Mg
   e. Thyroid function: TSH, and FT4 or FT1
   f. EKG as starvation may cause U waves, reduced QRS height, bradycardia; use of ipecac in bulimics has direct cardiotoxicity
   g. Serum carotene may be elevated in anorectics
   h. Serum amylase may be elevated with frequent vomiting or laxative use

V. Management

A. General approach to both conditions
1. Patients need close monitoring: even up to 2–3 times/wk for 4–6 wk
2. In many cases, family therapy is highly recommended
3. Depressive symptoms and suicidal ideation should be addressed in both bulimics and anoretics

    4. Many patients conceal or deny their problem and this often impacts on the therapeutic plan
    5. The primary care physician must consider physical problems associated with eating disorders
      a. Hypothyroidism
      b. Neurovegetative slowing
      c. Amenorrhea
      d. Upper GI bleeding from induced vomiting
      e. Akinetic colon
      f. Chronic diarrhea
    6. Care plan usually should involve the primary physician working in conjunction with the psychiatric team so as to avoid being drawn by the patient into a power struggle
    7. Inpatient care should be considered if there is
      a. Weight loss >30%
      b. Severe electrolyte or metabolic disturbance
      c. Suicidal ideation or psychotic behavior
      d. Severe binging and/or purging
      e. Family crisis
      f. Failure of outpatient psychiatric treatment to improve physical symptoms or signs
      g. Actual or imminent danger to the patient for medical reasons (e.g., severe vomiting with electrolyte balance)
B. **For bulimia care may include**
    1. Self-monitoring with record-keeping of foods consumed, eating times and degree of control when eating
    2. Focusing patient on aspects of functioning other than appearance
    3. Eating 3 or 4 regular, planned meals per day
    4. Counseling on coping with stress (rather than use of overeating) and recognizing precipitating causes of binges and/or impulsive behaviors
    5. Counseling tactics on stopping binges and purges
    6. Drug therapy may be helpful, especially when eating disorder is associated with depressive symptoms; this should be discussed with psychiatric team

V. **Referral to Psychiatrist for**
    A. Uncertainty of diagnosis or treatment
    B. Suspicion of other psychiatric disorder
    C. Evaluation of degree of severity of disorder
    D. Severe disease

References

1. American College of Physicians: Eating disorders: Anorexia nervosa and bulimia. Ann Intern Med 105:790–794, 1986.
2. D'Angelo LJ, Farrow J: Clinical problems in adolescent medicine. J Gen Intern Med 4:64–73, 1984.

Endocarditis Prophylaxis

I. **General Principles**

    A. Recommendations for prophylaxis are based on animal models, in vitro studies, and current clinical knowledge, not on controlled trials

    B. Most oral, dental, and upper respiratory procedures are considered low-risk, and prophylaxis in these instances is usually with a single drug, taken orally

    C. Some practitioners, however, recommend using IV or broader-spectrum coverage for even low-risk procedures when patients are at high risk

    D. If in doubt, consult with infectious disease specialist or cardiologist

II. **Recommendations for Adults**

    A. Prophylaxis for procedures listed below (II. D) is indicated for the following conditions, which are low risk unless otherwise noted

        1. Prosthetic valves: all types (high risk)

        2. Previous infective endocarditis (high risk)

        3. Surgically constructed systemic–pulmonary shunts (high risk)

        4. Congenital cardiac malformations except for

            a. Isolated secundum ASD

            b. A surgically repaired ASD, VSD or PDA with no residual murmur for more than 6 mo

        5. Hypertrophic obstructive cardiomyopathy (HOCM)

        6. Acquired valvular disorders before and after valvular repair

        7. Mitral valve prolapse (MVP) with valvular regurgitation

    B. **The following conditions do not need prophylaxis**

        1. Hearts without known pathology

        2. MVP without regurgitation

        3. Physiologic, functional, or innocent murmurs

        4. History of rheumatic fever without valvular disease

    C. **No clear guidelines** are available for the following

        1. MVP with valve thickening or redundancy (by echocardiogram), especially in men over 45 y/o

        2. Cardiac transplant recipients (risk is not yet defined)

    D. **Procedures for which prophylaxis is currently recommended**

        1. **Dental:** gingival/mucosal bleeding expected

        2. **Oral:** tonsillectomy, adenoidectomy

        3. **Respiratory:** rigid bronchoscopy and surgery involving respiratory mucosa

        4. **Upper GI tract:** variceal sclerotherapy, esophageal dilatation, surgery that involves intestinal mucosa

5. **Lower GI tract:** any surgery that involves intestinal mucosa
6. **Gallbladder** surgery
7. **GU:** cystoscopy, urethral dilatation, prostatic surgery
   a. Any GU surgery or catheterization **if UTI present**
8. **Ob-Gyn:** vaginal hysterectomy
   a. **Prophylaxis indicated in the presence of infection for** vaginal delivery, cesarean section, D&C, abortion, IUD removal or placement, sterilization
9. **Other: I & D** of abscesses

E. **Low-risk procedures not requiring prophylaxis**
   1. Injection of local anesthetic for dental care
   2. Flexible bronchoscopy with or without biopsy
   3. Intubation
   4. EGD with or without biopsy
   5. Sigmoidoscopy or colonoscopy with or without biopsy

F. **For selected patients**
   1. Some physicians prefer to cover patients who are at high risk for infective endocarditis even for low-risk procedures (listed above)
   2. If questions arise, consult with cardiologist or infectious disease specialist

III. **Recommended Drug Regimens**

A. **General approach**
   1. Patients at risk who have oral, dental, or upper respiratory tract procedures may be given antibiotics PO only; IV is optional
   2. First dose is given prior to procedure
   3. Second dose—whether PO, IV, or IM—is ½ initial dose and is given 6 hr after initial dose
   4. For some procedures, practitioners may wish to substitute other antibiotics, depending on the infectious agent likely to be present

B. **Dental, oral, and upper respiratory tract**
   1. **By PO route**
      a. Amoxicillin: 3 g, 1 hr before procedure; then 1.5 g, 6 hr after initial dose
      b. For penicillin-allergic patients
         i. Erythromycin ethylsuccinate: 800 mg, 2 hr before procedure; then 400 mg 6 hr after initial dose
            or
         ii. Erythromycin stearate: 1 g, 2 hr before procedure; then .5 g 6 hr after initial dose
            or
         iii. Clindamycin: 300 mg, 1 hr before procedure; then 150 mg, 6 hr after initial dose
   2. **By IV or IM routes** when preferred by practitioner
      a. Ampicillin: 2 g IV or IM, 30 min before procedure; then 1 g IV or IM, 6 hr after initial dose

       i. Amoxicillin, 1.5 g PO, may be substituted for second dose
- b. For penicillin-allergic patients
  - i. Clindamycin: 300 mg IV, 30 min before procedure, 150 mg IV (or PO), at 6 hr after initial dose
3. For broader coverage of procedures, when so preferred
  - a. Gentamicin: 1.5 mg/kg (up to 80 mg) IV, given with ampicillin 2 g 30 min before procedure
    - i. Repeat at 8 hr after initial dose
    - ii. Amoxicillin 1.5 g PO may be substituted at 6 hr, with omission of second dose of gentamicin
  - b. For penicillin-allergic patients
    - i. Vancomycin: 1 g IV over 1 hr (to avoid "red-man" syndrome), starting 1 hr before procedure
      - (a) No repeat necessary
- C. **For GI, GU, Ob-Gyn,** the following IV regimens are recommended
  1. Gentamicin: 1.5 mg/kg (up to 80 mg) IV, given with ampicillin 2 g, 30 min before procedure
     - a. Repeat at 8 hr after initial dose
     - b. Amoxicillin 1.5 g PO at 6 hr may be substituted, with omission of second dose of gentamicin
  2. For penicillin-allergic patients
     - a. Vancomycin: 1 g IV (must be administered over 1 hr) with gentamicin 1.5 mg/kg (up to 80 mg) IV or IM, 1 hr before procedure
       - i. May repeat at 8 hr
  3. Some practitioners prefer using **oral regimen** for patients at low-risk for endocarditis
     - a. Amoxicillin: 3 g, 1 hr before procedure; then 1.5 g, 6 hr after initial dose
- D. **Special considerations**
  1. Patients with severe renal insufficiency may need modification of regimens
  2. Patients at risk for endocarditis need perioperative coverage during open-heart surgery, mostly for staph species
- E. **Consultation** with an infectious disease specialist or cardiologist is helpful for
  1. Uncertainty of proper coverage for patient or procedure

Reference

Dajani AS, Bisno AL, Chung KJ, et al: Prevention of bacterial endocarditis: Recommendations by the American Heart Association. JAMA 264:2919–2922, 1990.

Esophageal Disorders

I. **Definition**

Heartburn and indigestion are lay terms often used to describe noncardiac recurrent retrosternal chest discomfort

II. **General Principles**

A. **General classification of causes**
1. **Reflux esophagitis**
   a. No strong association between documented reflux and patient symptoms
2. **Esophageal motility disorders**
   a. "Nutcracker" esophagus is caused by prolonged, powerful peristaltic contractions
   b. Esophageal spasm with diffuse simultaneous contractions
3. **Esophageal distention**
   a. Functional (e.g., from cold or hot liquids)
   b. Mechanical obstruction (e.g., achalasia, tumor)
B. An important aspect of the differential diagnosis is eliminating cardiac pain as a cause of the discomfort
1. Frequently this may be done by history and physical examination and/or a few simple investigations
2. In some cases, evaluation of a potential cardiac cause necessitates extensive testing

III. **Diagnostics**

A. **History** and **examination** in many people focus on eliminating cardiac and musculoskeletal causes
B. **History of suspected noncardiac causes**
1. Duration of pain and timing in relation to meals
2. Type of pain and radiation
3. Association with certain foods (citrus juices, coffee, tea)
4. Association with lying down or bending over (reflux)
5. Taste of acid in mouth
6. Relief by antacids
7. Vomiting, timing of vomiting
8. Dysphagia
9. Systemic symptoms: weight loss, anorexia
C. **Examination**
1. Neck evaluation for mass, lymphadenopathy
2. Palpation of chest for musculoskeletal tenderness
3. Cardiovascular and respiratory systems
4. Abdominal examination for masses and tenderness
5. Fecal occult blood test

D. **Laboratory data**
  1. Investigations once cardiac causes are eliminated
     a. CBC and differential
     b. Electrolytes (particularly if patient has been vomiting)
     c. Creatinine and BUN
     d. Liver function tests
  2. Further investigation
     a. Upper GI series for esophageal or gastric abnormality
     b. Upper GI endoscopy (EGD) for esophagitis, gastritis, or other abnormality
     c. Ultrasound scan of abdomen, if biliary colic suspected
     d. Barium swallow if dysphagia is primary complaint
  3. Specialist investigations for selected patients
     a. Diffuse spasm: manometric studies
     b. Nutcracker esophagus: manometric studies
     c. Reflux: ambulatory monitoring of intraesophageal pH or acid perfusion (Bernstein) test

IV. **Management**

  A. **General approach**
    1. For uncomplicated reflux symptoms, simple measures (see below for details) often resolve the problem
    2. Many practitioners try the following before further tests or referral to GI specialist
       a. Elevate head of bed with brick or piece of wood
       b. Avoid spicy foods and irritant beverages (coffee, tea, citric acids, chocolates)
       c. Avoid eating within 2–3 hours of bedtime
       d. Avoid lying down after meals
       e. Normalize weight
       f. Stop or reduce alcohol intake
       g. Stop smoking
       h. Avoid tight clothes

  B. **A trial of therapy** may be useful before referral
    1. Antacids
       a. Aluminum and magnesium hydroxide compounds
          i. Maalox TC or Mylanta II
             (a) 15 ml (1 tbs) q.i.d., 30 min after meals and q.h.s.
          ii. Gelusil
       b. Magnesium hydroxide compounds
          i. Milk of magnesia
       c. Aluminum hydroxide compounds
          i. Amphojel or Riopan
       d. Calcium carbonate compounds
          i. Tums
       e. Alginic compounds
          i. Gaviscon
    2. H_2 blockers (in alphabetical order):

      a. Cimetidine (Tagamet) 400 mg b.i.d.
      b. Famotidine (Pepcid) 20 mg b.i.d.
      c. Nizatidine (Axid) 150 mg b.i.d.
      d. Ranitidine (Zantac) 150 mg b.i.d.
   3. Other drugs
      a. Carafate (sucralfate) 1 g q.i.d.
         i. Take on an empty stomach
         ii. Avoid concurrent antacids
      b. Metoclopramide (Reglan) 10 mg t.i.d.
         i. Increases gastric emptying
         ii. Take 30 min before meals
         iii. Often used with delayed gastric emptying
      c. Omeprazole (Prilosec) 20–40 mg q.d.
         i. Expensive drug indicated for severe or refractory erosive esophagitis

C. **For uncertain diagnosis, complicated reflux (see below), or poor response** to therapy, consider one or both of the following
   1. Endoscopy may be preferred for pain evaluation because it allows for visualization and biopsy, as necessary
   2. Upper GI series
      a. Can detect functional or mechanical abnormality
      b. Often test of choice for dysphagia

D. **Complicated reflux** may include symptoms/signs of
   1. Vomiting and/or hematemesis
   2. Dysphagia
   3. Loss of appetite and/or significant weight loss
   4. Guaiac-positive stool
   5. Persistent pain or discomfort
   6. Fatigue and malaise
   7. Anemia or other abnormal laboratory tests
   8. Failure of trial of therapy to improve symptoms

V. **Referral to Gastroenterologist for**

   A. Uncertainty of diagnosis or treatment
   B. Suspected serious underlying disorder
   C. Complicated symptomatology
   D. Failure of simple medical therapies
   E. Recurrent or persistent symptoms
   F. Specialized studies or procedures

References

1. Editorial: Medical therapy for reflux esophagitis: 1986 and beyond. Ann Intern Med 104:112–114, 1986.
2. Hixson LJ, Kelley CL, Jones WN, Tuohy CD: Current trends in the pharmacotherapy for gastroesophageal reflux disease. Arch Intern Med 152:717–723, 1992.
3. Richter JE, Bradley LA, Castell DO: Esophageal chest pain: Current controversies in pathogenesis, diagnosis, and therapy. Ann Intern Med 110:66–78, 1989.

G

Gallstones and Gallbladder Disease

I. **General Principles**

   A. In industrialized countries, most gallstones (80%) are cholesterol stones

   B. Prevalence of all stones is estimated at 10% of the population

   C. Incidence of gallstones increases with

     1. Age

     2. Obesity

     3. Estrogens such as birth control pill, pregnancy, postmenopausal replacement

     4. Ileal dysfunction such as with inflammatory bowel diseases, intestinal bypass surgery

     5. Impaired emptying of gallbladder, including fasting, TPN, pregnancy, and, possibly, liquid diets

     6. Certain drugs such as cholestyramine, colestipol

     7. Sickle-cell disease

   D. Most gallstones (60–80%) are asymptomatic and are found coincidentally by imaging tests

II. **Diagnostics**

   A. **History**

     1. Presence of symptoms

       a. Biliary colic

       b. Upper right quadrant or epigastric pain

       c. Pain to shoulder or into back

       d. Postprandial or indigestion-type discomfort

     2. History of pancreatitis or acute cholecystitis

     3. Episodes of fever, nausea, vomiting, intermittent jaundice, acholic stools, or dark urine

     4. Medications

     5. Previous surgery

     6. Diet and eating habits

   B. **Examination** (frequently unremarkable)

     1. Sclera for icterus

     2. Abdominal palpation for masses, tenderness (Murphy's sign)

   C. **Laboratory data**

     1. **For selected patients**

       a. CBC and differential for evaluation of cholecystitis (or if chronic hemolysis suspected)

       b. LFTs (aminotransferases, bilirubin, alkaline phosphatase) to determine degree of liver dysfunction

    c. Amylase/lipase if pancreatitis suspected

    d. Urinalysis to determine if direct bilirubin present

2. **Imaging tests**

    a. Ultrasound scan

        i. Accuracy in detecting gallstones

           (a) Sensitivity: 90–95%

           (b) Specificity: 94–98%

       ii. Patient should fast prior to test for at least 6 hr

      iii. Findings compatible with acute cholecystitis

           (a) Stones/sludge

           (b) Gallbladder (GB) wall >5 mm in thickness

           (c) Murphy's sign elicited with sonogram

           (d) GB enlargement and round-shaped GB

    b. Technetium HIDA nuclear scan

        i. Tests for cystic duct patency and GB motility

       ii. Usually used when acute cholecystitis is clinically suspected

      iii. Patient fasts for 2–4 hr before study

      iv. Accuracy for detecting acute cholecystitis

           (a) Sensitivity: 95–97%

           (b) Specificity: 90–97%

       v. Accuracy for detecting chronic cholecystitis

           (a) Sensitivity: 45%

           (b) Specificity: 90%

      vi. Finding compatible with acute cholecystitis is nonvisualization

      vii. Finding compatible for chronic cholecystitis is that GB takes >1 hr to be visualized

III. **Management**

A. **Asymptomatic** gallstones do not require active intervention but general advice may include

1. Avoid rapid weight reduction

2. Use of different medications, if appropriate

3. Seek medical attention if symptoms develop

B. **Symptomatic** gallstones

1. **Nonsurgical** approaches

    a. **Oral bile acids**

        i. 10–15% of patients meet criteria for receiving bile acids

       ii. Usual Rx is for 1–2 yr

      iii. Refer to gastroenterologist for initiating treatment

      iv. For **radiolucent stones** <15 mm in diameter in functioning GB, consider

           (a) Ursodeoxycholic acid (Ursidiol), 10–13 mg/kg q.d.

           (b) Chenodeoxycholic acid (Chenodiol), 15 mg/kg q.d.

               (i) Usual initial dose is 250 mg b.i.d.

      v. Dissolves up to 60% of stones

      vi. Most successful in stones ≤**5 mm** in diameter and **floating**

      vii. Monitor with

         (a) Ultrasound periodically to check for recurrence after treatment discontinued

         (b) LFTs

  b. **Lithotripsy** (ESWL)

      i. 10–15% of patients meet criteria for receiving lithotripsy

      ii. For **radiolucent** stones, best with single stone

      iii. Side effects from passage of stone fragments

         (a) Pancreatitis (1–2%)

         (b) Cholecystitis (1%)

         (c) Emergency ERCP or cholecystectomy (<5%)

      iv. Monitor with ultrasound to check for recurrence

  c. **Contact dissolution**

      i. Still experimental therapy

      ii. For patients with open cystic duct, radiolucent stone, and GB attached to liver bed

      iii. Requires inpatient therapy for 3–4 d

      iv. Annual recurrence rate may be up to 30%

2. **Surgical** approaches

  a. **Laparoscopic cholecystectomy**

      i. Most patients are eligible for this procedure

      ii. Inpatient stay 1–2 d

      iii. Return to normal daily activities 1–2 wk

      iv. Mortality <1%

      v. Complication rate <5%

         (a) Bile duct injury: 0.3–0.5%

      vi. Open cholecystectomy needed in 4–5% of patients

      vii. Patients often not eligible if they have

         (a) Acute cholecystitis or pancreatitis

         (b) Likelihood of adhesions in surgical field

  b. Open cholecystectomy is the traditional approach

IV. **Referral to a Gastroenterologist or General Surgeon for Symptomatic Gallstones**

References

1. American College of Physicians: How to study the gallbladder. Ann Intern Med 109:752–754, 1988
2. Paumgartner G, Sauerbruch T: Gallstones: Pathogenesis. Lancet 338:1117–1121, 1991.
3. Sauerbruch T, Paumgartner G: Gallbladder stones: Management. Lancet 338:1121–1124, 1991.

Gout

I. Definition

Gout is a crystal-induced arthropathy associated with monosodium urate crystals

II. General Principles

A. Prevalence of gout is about 275 cases/100,000 persons (.00275%)
B. Manifestations of hyperuricemia may be classified as
   1. Asymptomatic
   2. Acute gouty arthritis
   3. Tophaceous gout
   4. Gouty renal impairment (nephropathy)
   5. Renal uric acid calculi
C. Most patients with hyperuricemia have inappropriately low renal excretion rates of uric acid
   1. A small percentage of patients (10–15%) are overproducers of uric acid, defined as >600 mg of urinary uric acid (in men) per 24 hr while on a purine free diet (or >750 mg/24 hr on a regular diet)
D. Drugs and substances that increase serum uric acid
   1. Diuretics such as thiazides and loop compounds
   2. Alcohol
   3. Nicotinic acid
   4. Chemotherapeutic agents

III. Diagnostics

A. **History**
   1. Characteristics of acute attacks
      a. Abrupt onset
      b. Extreme tenderness of joint(s)
   2. Joints affected are often one or more of
      a. Metatarsophalangeal (MTP) of big toe
      b. Knee
      c. Ankle
      d. Wrist
      e. Finger
   3. Age at onset and intervals (months, years) between attacks
   4. Duration of episodes is often 3–10 d
   5. Previous investigations and treatments
   6. History of tophi or renal calculi
   7. Medications
B. **Examination**
   1. Warm, red, swollen, and extremely tender joint in acute stages
   2. Search for tophaceous deposits

C. **Laboratory data**
1. Serum urate levels
    a. Normal levels do not exclude gout
2. **Examination of joint fluid**
    a. Rod- or needle-shaped crystals
        i. Intra- or extracellular
        ii. Best seen with polarized microscope as negatively birefringent crystals
    b. Synovial fluid examination
        i. White cell count usually 2000–20,000 cells/mm³ but may be as high as 100,000 cells
        ii. Neutrophils predominate
        iii. Viscosity
3. Creatinine and BUN
D. **Further investigations**
1. CBC and differential if infection suspected
2. Urinalysis if renal disease suspected or patient has history of renal colic or stones
3. X-rays of affected joints
4. Serum glucose if diabetes suspected
5. 24-hr urine collection for creatinine and uric acid
    a. Excretion of urate >750 mg/24 hr on regular diet indicates overproduction of uric acid
    b. Test should be used when result will affect treatment (e.g., whether to start allopurinol)
6. SGOT/SGPT if hepatic disease suspected as precipitant of gout

IV. **Management**

A. **General approach**
1. With **asymptomatic hyperuricemia,** treatment is not necessary
    a. Some patients may benefit from treatment with allopurinol if 24-hr urine secretion of uric acid >1100 mg/d
2. **Indications for lowering serum urate**
    a. Tophaceous gout
    b. Renal disease or stone formation
    c. Frequent gouty attacks
3. **When beginning therapy with allopurinol** or uricosuric drug
    a. Begin prophylactic colchicine (0.5–1.2 mg q.d.) to avoid precipitating acute gout
    b. Patient with tophaceous gout may need 6–12 mo of prophylaxis to avoid acute gout
    c. Patients who cannot take colchicine can be given low- to moderate-dose NSAID therapy
B. **Pharmacologic therapy**
1. **Acute gout**
    a. **NSAID of choice**
        i. Given in full therapeutic dosage initially and tapered off as attack resolves (usually 7–10 d)

        ii. Taken with food to reduce GI side effects

       iii. Commonly used NSAIDs

          (a) Indomethacin: 50 mg t.i.d.–q.i.d.

          (b) Naproxen: 250 mg t.i.d., after taking initial loading dose of 750 mg

          (c) Sulindac: 200 mg b.i.d.

b. Colchicine

    i. 0.5–1.2 mg initially, then 0.5–1.2 mg q 2 hr until pain relief or GI toxicity (diarrhea, nausea) occurs, or reach maximum dosage

    ii. Maximum dose is 4–8 mg in 24 hr

    iii. Patient should begin therapy at earliest symptoms of gouty attack

    iv. Once attack subsides, further colchicine is often not needed for at least 7 d (due to its long half-life)

    v. Lower doses may be necessary in persons with renal insufficiency or hepatic disease or in the elderly

    vi. Avoid in patients with renal failure

c. Corticosteroids

    i. Prednisone (or equivalent) at 30 mg q.d., tapering as attack resolves

    ii. Colchicine or NSAID often needed while tapering steroid to prevent relapse of attack

2. **For recurrent gout:** treatment and/or prophylaxis

a. NSAIDs

    i. Patients should begin medication, in doses listed above, at the earliest symptom of acute gout

    ii. Use low to moderate doses to protect against acute exacerbation when patient begins allopurinol or probenecid

b. Colchicine

    i. For chronic prophylaxis: 0.5–0.6 mg q.d.–b.i.d., using lowest possible dose to control attacks

    ii. If allopurinol or probenecid therapy is started, continue daily dose for 6–12 mo

c. Allopurinol (100–800 mg q.d.)

    i. Low dose at 100 mg q.d. may be effective

    ii. Most persons have maintenance therapy of 300 mg q.d.

    iii. Use lowest effective dose

    iv. Reduce dose in patients with renal insufficiency

    v. Drug of choice for persons who

      (a) Have overexcretion of urate in urine

      (b) Have renal disease or tophaceous gout

      (c) Are on chronic aspirin therapy

      (d) Have uric acid renal stone

    vi. Begin prophylaxis with colchicine (or NSAID) to avoid precipitating acute gout

    d. **Probenecid**
      i. Patient should not have overexcretion of urate in urine
      ii. Starting dose is 250 mg b.i.d. for 1 wk, then 500 mg b.i.d. with additional increases, if necessary
      iii. Maximum dose is 2 g/d
      iv. Increase fluid intake for at least first few mo of therapy
      v. Not effective when creatinine clearance is <35 ml/min
      vi. Begin prophylaxis with colchicine (or NSAID) to avoid precipitating acute gout

C. **Monitoring**
  1. Periodic monitoring includes
    a. Serum urate and creatinine, BUN when urate-lowering drugs are used
    b. CBC for those on allopurinol and colchicine (maintenance) treatment

V. **Referral to Rheumatologist for**

A. Uncertainty of diagnosis or treatment
B. Monitoring therapy
C. Complications of gout or hyperuricemia

References

1. American College of Rheumatology: Guidelines for Reviewers of Rheumatic Disease Care. ACR, 1989, pp 6–7.
2. American Rheumatism Association: Dictionary of the Rheumatic Disease. Vol. II: Diagnostic Testing. ARA, 1985, pp 88–91.
3. Arthritis Foundation: Primer on Rheumatic Diseases, 9th ed. Atlanta, Arthritis Foundation, 1988, pp 195–207.

Gynecologic Bleeding

I. **General Principles**

A. Most causes of gynecologic bleeding are benign but cancer is not infrequent
  1. Cervical cancer incidence is about 17,000 cases/yr
  2. Uterine cancer incidence is about 34,000 cases/yr
B. Other causes of genital bleeding include
  1. Dysfunctional bleeding such as estrogen breakthrough or withdrawal
  2. Disease of the genital tract
    a. Vaginal: exterior or interior laceration or lesion
    b. Cervix: polyp
    c. Uterus/endometrium: leiomyoma, polyp

3. Pregnancy
    a. Threatened or inevitable abortion
    b. Ectopic
4. Other (rare causes)
    a. Leukemia or bleeding disorder
    b. Thrombocytopenia
    c. Thyroid disease

II. **Diagnostics**

A. **History includes**

1. Gynecologic history including infections and/or abnormal discharge as well as characteristics of discharge (itchy, aromatic)
2. Menstrual history: menarche, menopause, cycle length, days bleeding, date of last "normal" menstrual bleed
3. Reproductive history
4. Contraceptive use: type, duration, previous history
5. Coital history: deep or superficial dyspareunia, partner history(ies)
6. Endometrial cancer risks which include
    a. Hypertension
    b. Estrogen replacement therapy
    c. Nulliparity
    d. Obesity
    e. Diabetes mellitus
7. DES exposure in utero (increases risk of vaginal cancer)
8. Type and heaviness of bleeding (e.g., how many pads/d needed) including
    a. Spotting or steady bleeding
    b. Clots or fresh blood

B. **Full examination includes**

1. Abdominal exam for masses
2. Examination of perineum, vagina and cervix
    a. Include visualization and digital palpation
3. Rectal

C. **Initial investigations for selected patients**

1. Urine pregnancy test if the woman is premenopausal
2. Pap smear
3. Cultures: chlamydia, gonococcus
4. Wet mount and potassium hydroxide preparations
5. Hemoglobin/hematocrit if bleeding is heavy

D. **For patients who have no discernible cause for bleeding, consider**

1. Thyroid study: TSH and FT4 or FTI
2. Bleeding time
3. Platelets
4. Renal function tests (uremia as a cause of platelet dysfunction)

III. **Management**

  A. **General approach**
    1. If **vaginitis and/or abnormal discharge noted**
      a. Evaluate wet mount and KOH preparation, and send vaginal cultures, if indicated
      b. See chapter on STD for details of treatment
      c. Check pregnancy test; if pregnant, consult gynecologist for appropriate treatment
    2. If patient **pregnant and**
      a. **Ectopic pregnancy** suspected, arrange emergency pelvic ultrasound and/or **refer to emergency care immediately**
      b. Cervical os closed in an intrauterine pregnancy
        i. Likely threatened abortion
          • Advise bedrest and refer to Ob/Gyn follow-up
      c. Cervical os open
        i. Likely inevitable abortion
          • Refer to Ob/Gyn
    3. If mass palpated during abdominal or pelvic exam
      a. Check pregnancy test
      b. Request ultrasound exam
      c. Refer to gynecologist for evaluation

IV. **Referral to a Gynecologist for**

  A. Further evaluation of abnormal genital bleeding
  B. Post menopausal bleeding

Reference

Cowan BD, Morrison JC: Current Concepts: Management of abnormal genital bleeding in girls and women. N Engl J Med 324:1710–1715, 1991.

H

Headache

I. General Principles

    A. Less than 1% of headaches are caused by potentially dangerous problems

    B. Most headaches (80%) are categorized as due to muscular tension

    C. An estimated 10–20% of people suffer from recurrent migrainous headaches

    D. Prevalence of headaches decreases with age

    E. A person older than 55 yr, with new onset of headaches, should be carefully evaluated for serious underlying cause

II. General Classification of Headaches (Selected Listing)

    A. Inflammatory or infectious
        1. Temporal arteritis
        2. Intracranial infection/abscess
        3. Sinusitis and other ENT problems
        4. Temporomandibular joint pain

    B. Muscular or tension
        1. Stress
        2. Eye strain from refractory error

    C. Vascular
        1. Migraine
        2. Cluster
        3. Hypertensive
        4. Exertional or coital

    D. Mass lesions
        1. Infections
        2. Neoplastic
            a. Primary
            b. Secondary

    E. Mixed/other
        1. Aspects usually of vascular and muscular
        2. Medications induced
        3. Medication withdrawal (including from headache Rx)

III. Characteristics of Migraine Headaches

    A. Common migraine (80–85% of migraines)
        1. Usually unilateral, throbbing headache with variable prodromal symptoms
        2. Occasionally bilateral
        3. Often associated with noise and photophobia
        4. Prodrome is often mood or GI upset
        5. Headache may become generalized

    6. Onset and duration may be hours or days

    7. Frequently with nausea, vomiting

    8. No neurologic symptoms

B. **Classic migraine (15–20%)**

    1. Unilateral onset with prodromal symptoms

    2. Prodromes often visual or minor sensory

    3. Often with anorexia, nausea, and photophobia

    4. Usually lasts 6–12 hr

    5. Frequent family history of same

C. **Complicated migraine**

    1. As above but neurological alteration may be severe

IV. **Characteristics of Tension Headache**

A. Tight or constrictive achiness

B. Often suboccipital or frontal/occipital (hatband distribution)

C. Duration may be over hours or many days

D. Associated with persistent tenseness of neck and shoulder muscles

E. May be associated with stress at home, at work, or in social sphere

V. **Characteristics of Cluster Headaches**

A. Rapid onset of brief, often sharp unilateral head pain, usually orbital or retroorbital pain of 20–30 min duration

B. Frequently with facial redness, eye watering, and rhinorrhea

C. A minority (20%) may have ptosis or miosis

D. Patients often have smoking or heavy alcohol use history

VI. **Characteristics of Temporal Arteritis**

A. Almost always in older (>55 y/o) patients

B. Women are much more commonly affected than men

C. Temporal pain and scalp tenderness

D. Jaw claudication

E. Visual dimming on affected side (often a late and ominous sign)

F. Pulseless, hard, tender temporal artery

G. Often associated with systemic signs and/or polymyalgia rheumatica

H. Raised ESR

VII. **Diagnostics**

A. **History**

    1. Age at onset of headaches

    2. Recurrence rate

    3. Duration and severity of symptoms

    4. Characteristics of headache

    5. Precipitating stimuli such as emotions, foods, and odors

    6. Presence of aura or flickering lights

    7. Association with sinus difficulties, ear pain, or jaw pain

      8. Presence of visual dimming, jaw claudication, temporal tenderness
      9. Family history of migraine headaches

B. Examination
    1. General observation of mental status and cognition
    2. Fundal and visual assessment
    3. Neurological examination
    4. Eliciting areas of sinus or facial tenderness
    5. Temporal artery palpation in older persons
    6. Auscultation for bruits over orbit
    7. Neck musculature tenderness
    8. Range of movement of neck

C. Laboratory data
    1. For selected patients, depending on clinical evaluation
      a. CBC and differential
      b. ESR to evaluate for temporal arteritis, usually in older patients
      c. Sinus films and/or sinus CT scan if sinus disease suspected
         • See chapter on "Sinusitis" for details
      d. CT of head is considered when there is
         i. Abnormal neurological examination
         ii. Recent significant change in characteristics of chronic headache
         iii. New onset after age 40 y/o
         iv. Orbital bruit
         v. Other warning signs of serious disorder (see below)
      e. Temporal artery biopsy if arteritis suspected by history or examination

VIII. Management

A. General approach
    1. If headache is thought to have potentially dangerous underlying cause, request appropriate evaluations and refer urgently
      a. If **temporal arteritis** seems likely, before or after ESR result, treat immediately with high-dose steroids (60–80 mg) and obtain biopsy as soon as possible
      b. If hypertension is suspected cause of headache, evaluate as per hypertensive emergency
         • See chapter on "Hypertension: Urgent and Emergent"
      c. **Warning signs of serious disorder**
         i. New asymmetric neurologic deficits
         ii. Transient losses of vision
         iii. Headaches first beginning after age 55
         iv. Significant worsening of previously stable headaches
         v. Most severe headache patient has ever had
         vi. Encephalitic or meningitic signs or symptoms
         vii. History of cancer or other systemic disorder
         viii. History of certain infectious diseases (e.g., HIV, TB)
         ix. Finding of orbital bruit

B. **Benign recurrent headaches**
1. Advise patient to avoid triggers (e.g., chocolates, red wine, lack of sleep, irregular eating habits)
2. Avoid, whenever possible, prescribing habit-forming drugs such as barbiturates, benzodiazepines, and narcotic analgesics
3. Relaxation therapy, aerobic exercise, and/or biofeedback may be useful
4. Educate patient on effects of stress, including jaw clenching, neck and upper back strain
5. Reassure patient about benign nature of headache

C. **Migraine headaches**
1. **For acute or abortive treatment,** consider
   a. Naproxen: 500 mg b.i.d.; effective for some patients
   b. Propranolol: 40–120 mg at onset of attack may be useful for some patients
   c. Ergotamine may be given
      i. Sublingually or orally, 1–2 mg, q 30 min, up to 6 mg/d or 10 mg/wk
      ii. By suppository, 2 mg initially, repeat in 1 hr up to 4 mg per attack or 10 mg/wk
   d. Dihydroergotamine
      i. Can be given as 0.5 mg IV or 1 mg IM at the beginning of the headache
      ii. Repeated q 8 hr if headache continues
   e. Considerations
      i. Ergotamine can be given with caffeine (e.g., Cafergot) and/or with an antiemetic (e.g., metoclopramide, 10 mg PO or IM)
      ii. Adverse effects of ergotamine
         (a) May be habit-forming
         (b) May cause rebound headaches when used frequently
      iii. Contraindications for use of ergotamine
         (a) Coronary and peripheral artery disease
         (b) Renal and hepatic failure
         (c) Hypertension
         (d) Pregnancy
         (e) Complicated migraine
      iv. A new drug, sumatriptan (100 mg PO, repeated at 2 hr if necessary) may soon be available in U.S. and appears to be effective in relieving acute migraines
2. **Prophylaxis** for severe frequent headaches (i.e., 2–4/mo) or for when therapies for acute attacks are inadequate
   a. Propranolol
      i. May be started at 10–20 mg b.i.d., up to 160–240 mg/d (in divided doses)
      ii. Sustained-release preparation is also available at an initial dose of 80 mg q.d., increasing to 160–240 mg/d

           iii. Other beta blockers (e.g., timolol, nadolol, atenolol) may be substituted

      b. Verapamil

          i. 180 SR, q.d., up to 360 mg by SR or divided doses

          ii. Other calcium channel blocker may be substituted

      c. Amitriptyline

          i. 10 or 25 mg q.h.s., increasing slowly as needed and as tolerated, up to 150 mg q.h.s.

D. Cluster headaches

1. Acute or abortive therapy
   a. Ergotamine
      i. 1–2 mg at onset of or prior to usual time of attack may help
      ii. Can increase to 4 mg/d
   b. Simple analgesic of choice (e.g., Tylenol, aspirin) may be all that is needed in some cases
2. Prophylaxis
   a. Methysergide (4–8 mg q.d.)
      i. Trial of therapy is usually 3 wk
      ii. Must be discontinued for 1 mo after every 6 mo of use
   b. Verapamil (180–360 mg/d by SR or divided doses)
   c. Prednisone (20–40 mg q.d. tapered over 3 wk)
      i. May interfere with cycle of cluster headaches

E. Tension headaches

1. General education on stress reduction and relaxation and exercise may be of great assistance
2. Consider advice on hot baths and neck or back massage
3. Temporary relief may sometimes be achieved with NSAIDs or muscle relaxants, although these do not address the underlying problem and should not be used on constant basis

IX. Referral to Neurologist for

A. Uncertainty of diagnosis or treatment
B. Suspected serious neurologic or underlying disease
C. Headaches recalcitrant to medical therapies listed above
D. Patient reassurance

References

1. Kumar KL, Cooney TG: Vascular headache. J Gen Intern Med 3:384–395, 1988.
2. Lance JW: Treatment of migraine. Lancet 339:1207–1209, 1992.
3. Smith MJ, Jensen NM: The severity model of chronic headache. J Gen Intern Med 3:396–409, 1988.

Head and Neck Cancer

I. **General Principles**

   A. Peak incidence occurs in 50–60 y/o with men outnumbering women 3 to 1
   B. Almost all cancers (95%) are squamous
   C. Spread occurs to local nodes, lung, bone, and liver
   D. Risk factors for squamous cell cancer of the head and neck, by affected areas
      1. **Oral cavity, hypopharynx, and oropharynx:** alcohol, tobacco, Betel nut juice
      2. **Larynx:** tobacco, alcohol, asbestos, exposure to metal processing byproducts
      3. **Nasal cavity:** nickel, chromium, exposure to wood and leather-working byproducts
      4. **Sinuses:** as for nasal cavity
   E. Stages are generally classified as
      1. I and II: small primary tumors without node involvement or distant spread; prognosis is good
      2. III and above: large tumors or spread to lymph nodes or distant sites

II. **Diagnostics**

   A. **History** should raise suspicion if patients have
      1. Persistent mouth ulcers or local pain
      2. Dentures that have become poorly fitting
      3. Hoarseness >3–6 wk
      4. Sore throat >3–6 wk with no response to antibiotics
      5. Persistent sinusitis or bloody discharge from nose
   B. **Examination**
      1. Oral leukoplakia (white patches)
      2. Oral erythroplakia (velvety red patches)
      3. Oral ulcers that persist
      4. Loosening tooth or teeth
      5. Cheek swelling or proptosis
      6. Otitis media in an adult
      7. Neck masses and lymph node enlargement
   C. **Laboratory data**
      1. For selected patients, depending on clinical evaluation
         a. Indirect laryngoscopy if mouth or throat symptoms
         b. Biopsy for leukoplakia or erythroplakia
         c. CXR
         d. Sinus films if sinus symptoms
         e. Thyroid scan for low neck masses
         f. CBC
         g. Liver function tests

2. Imaging studies
   a. CT/MRI roles are not specifically defined
   b. Refer to ENT physician for guidance

D. **For asymptomatic enlarged cervical lymph node**
   1. Do not order biopsy unless evaluation yields no diagnosis of primary lesion
   2. General order of evaluation
      a. Palpate base of tongue with gloved finger
      b. Attempt indirect laryngoscopy
      c. Request CXR
      d. Sinus films or thyroid scan if symptoms or signs raise suspicion
      e. Refer for panendoscopy
      f. Open biopsy of node (and/or neck dissection) if primary still not found

III. **Management**

   A. **General approach**
      1. Treatment options
         a. Removal and/or dissection
         b. Reconstruction
         c. Radiation
      2. Patients should have dental examination prior to radiation therapy

   B. **Following dissection and/or radiation treatment**
      1. Monitor for recurrence (usually within 3 yr)
      2. Check for second primary (20% of those cured)
      3. In patients with disfigurement or dysfunction, be aware of depressive and suicidal symptoms
      4. Monitor thyroid function (hypothyroidism from radiation)
      5. Advise on stopping cigarettes
         a. Patients who continue smoking have up to 40–60% chance of developing a second primary cancer
      6. Patient may need treatment for xerostomia

IV. **Referral to Head and Neck Specialist for**

   A. Uncertainty of diagnosis or diagnostic procedures
   B. Evaluation of undiagnosed asymptomatic lymph node enlargement

Reference

Jacobs J: The internist in the management of head and neck cancer. Ann Intern Med 113:771–778, 1990.

Hirsutism

I. Definition

Hirsutism in women is defined as excess body hair

II. General Principles

A. Hirsutism can be the precursor to, but is different from, virilization, which is masculinization of features
B. Between $1/6$ to $1/3$ of normal women have hair on their face, chest or breast, or lower abdomen
C. In a woman, about half of daily testosterone comes from the adrenals and half from the ovaries
D. Androgen excess can be classified
   1. **Adrenal:** Cushing's syndrome, congenital adrenal hyperplasias, malignancy
   2. **Ovarian:** polycystic ovaries (PCO), tumors, insulin resistance (variant of PCO), malignancy
   3. **Combined** ovarian and adrenal: idiopathic hirsutism
   4. **Medications:** anabolic steroids, birth control pills, minoxidil, phenytoin, glucocorticoids, cyclosporine

III. Diagnostics

A. **History**
   1. Age of onset
      a. Peripubertal suggests idiopathic or congenital adrenal hyperplasias
   2. Progression of increased hair growth: rapid (e.g., tumor) or slow (e.g., PCO)
   3. Family history for adrenal disorder or idiopathic hirsutism
   4. Drug history, especially from athletes, body builders
   5. Menstrual cycle, especially regularity
   6. Symptoms of virilization
      a. Frontal baldness
      b. Deepening of voice
      c. Cliteromegaly
      d. Increased facial or body acne
      e. Change toward male body habitus, especially of shoulder and pelvic girdle muscles
B. **Examination**
   1. Amount of hair and distribution: upper back, shoulders, sternum, and upper abdomen are abnormal
   2. Signs of Cushing's syndrome such as striae, fat distribution, hypertension
   3. Signs of insulin resistance such as acanthosis nigricans
   4. Drug-induced hirsutism, including widespread lanugo hair
   5. Pelvic examination for

a. Masses
b. Clitoral enlargement
6. Signs of virilization as listed above

C. **Laboratory data**
  1. If patient has **regular menses,** consider
     a. Serum total testosterone
        i. If testosterone is very high (>200 ng/dl), consider
           (a) CT scan of abdomen: for adrenal neoplasm
           (b) Pelvic ultrasound: for pelvic tumor
     b. Serum dehydroepiandrosterone sulfate (DHEA) levels
        i. Very high levels suggest adrenal neoplasm
        ii. May also be elevated in PCO, idiopathic hirsutism, or with ovarian tumors
     c. Serum 17-hydroxyprogesterone levels: taken once between 7 and 9 a.m.
        i. For congenital adrenal hyperplasias
        ii. Often done with cosyntropin stimulation for better accuracy
  2. If patient has **irregular menses,** consider
     a. Serum testosterone with further investigation if >200 ng/dl, as above
     b. Serum 17-hydroxyprogesterone levels, as above
     c. Serum DHEA sulfate or DHEA levels
     d. Serum prolactin level
  3. **For selected patients,** depending on clinical evaluation
     a. Urinary free cortisol if Cushing's syndrome suspected
     b. LH/FSH ratio: ≥3:1 is consistent with PCO
     c. Serum insulin levels to glucose load
        i. If insulin resistance (PCO) suspected
        ii. Refer to an endocrinologist prior to doing test
     d. Ovarian and adrenal vein catheterization
        i. If testosterone level is high without obvious cause
        ii. Refer to endocrinologist before doing test

IV. **Management**
  A. Specific medical or surgical treatment follows from diagnosis; refer or consult as appropriate
  B. Most diagnoses are of idiopathic causes and PCO
     1. Treatment regimens may include use of
        a. Spironolactone
        b. Combined oral contraceptives
  C. **Note:** if patient becomes ovulatory as a result of treatment, then she needs contraception if pregnancy is not desired
  D. If uncertain of work-up or treatment at any time, refer to or seek advice from an endocrinologist or specialist
  E. With treatment of underlying cause for hirsutism, excess hair may resolve, become less coarse, or lighten
     1. This may be a slow process (i.e., >6 mo)
  F. **Cosmetic**

1. Bleaching, hair removal techniques (electrolysis), or shaving may help
   a. Shaving does not cause hair to grow more rapidly
2. Other hair removal techniques include waxing and chemical removal
   a. These do not permanently remove hair and must be repeated periodically
G. Virilization changes (e.g., clitoromegaly) are often not reversible

V. **Referral to an Endocrinologist or Gynecologist for**
   A. Uncertainty of diagnosis and treatment
   B. Further evaluation after initial assessment
   C. Suspected or documented endocrine disease
   D. Suspected or documented adrenal or ovarian tumor

Reference

Rittmaster RS, Loriaux DL: Hirsutism. Ann Intern Med 106:95–107, 1987.

Hormone Replacement Therapy

I. **General Principles**
   A. Menopause occurs, on average, at age 50
   B. Approximately 30 million women in the U.S. are postmenopausal
   C. **Reduction in endogenous estrogen may precipitate** any or all of
      1. Acceleration of cardiovascular disease
      2. Symptoms of menopause
         a. Vasomotor effects (hot flashes)
         b. Psychological upset (mood swings, depression)
      3. Vaginal atrophy
         a. Vaginitis
         b. Dyspareunia
         c. Dysuria
      4. Aging of the skin
   D. **Indications for estrogen replacement therapy**
      1. Prevention and/or treatment of osteoporosis
      2. Risk reduction for cardiovascular disease
      3. Premature ovarian failure
      4. Symptoms of vasomotor disturbances in postmenopausal period
      5. Symptoms of vaginal atrophy
      6. Hypogonadism because of hypothalamic–pituitary failure
      7. Oophorectomy/castration in a premenopausal woman
   E. **Risks of estrogen replacement**
      1. Increased risk of endometrial hyperplasia and endometrial cancer (primarily with unopposed estrogens)

2. Risk of breast cancer
3. Increased incidence and/or severity of migraine headaches
4. Increased risk of thromboembolic disease

F. **Contraindications and precautions** for replacement therapy
1. **General contraindications**
   a. Recent myocardial infarction
   b. Cerebrovascular disease (stroke or TIAs)
   c. Thromboembolic disease
   d. Breast or endometrial cancer
   e. Hepatic dysfunction (severe)
   f. Undiagnosed vaginal bleeding
2. **Relative contraindications**
   a. Seizure disorders
   b. Uterine leiomyomas
   c. Familial hyperlipidemia
   d. Migraines
   e. Deep thrombophlebitis
   f. Endometriosis
   g. Gallbladder disease
   h. Hypertension

II. **Diagnostics**

A. **History:** discussion of above symptoms, risks, and contraindications

B. **Examination**
1. Blood pressure measurement
2. Breast and pelvic examination

C. **Laboratory data**
1. **Routine**
   a. Cervical smear (every 1–3 yr)
   b. Mammography (as indicated by age and risk factors)
2. **For selected patients**
   a. Endometrial biopsy
      i. Usually indicated if dysfunctional uterine bleeding is suspected
      ii. Should be considered prior to therapy in women with higher risks of endometrial cancer
         (a) Hypertensive, obese women
         (b) Diabetics
   b. FSH and LH (optional) if menopause is in question
   c. Baseline cholesterol and lipid level
      i. May alter because of progestin, with HDL decreasing and LDL increasing

III. **Management**

A. **General approach**
1. Estrogen therapy is usually given in cycles
2. The lowest dose to control symptoms is used
3. Women should be advised of the potential for withdrawal bleeding during cycle of replacement therapy
4. Currently there is wide variability of dosage regimens
   a. Progestins may be given concurrently with estrogens or for part of the estrogen replacement cycle

      b. Dosages of estrogens and progestins vary widely; the lowest effective dose of both drugs is recommended

   5. Discuss possible risks of taking HRT while continuing tobacco use, when appropriate

B. Pharmacologic therapy

   1. Estrogen alone

     a. Not usually used in women with intact endometrium due to increased risk of endometrial cancer

     b. Estrogens can be given intravaginally for atrophic vaginitis or urethritis, but this will not act as hormone replacement

        i. 1 applicator q.d., for 2 wk

        ii. Then ½ applicator q.d., for 2 wk

        iii. Then 1 applicator, 1–3 ×/wk for maintenance

   2. **General approach to cyclical therapy**

     a. Progestin may be given for 12–14 d of a monthly cycle with estrogen (cyclical)

         or

     b. Progestin and estrogen may be given daily (continuous)

        i. Dose of progestin is usually lower for this method

     c. Example of cyclical therapy

        i. Conjugated estrogen (Premarin): 0.625 mg PO, on days 1–25, every month

        ii. Medroxyprogesterone (Provera): 5–10 mg on days 16–25, every month

        iii. Withdrawal bleeding begins 3–7 days after discontinuation of Premarin/Provera

     d. An example of continuous therapy

        i. Conjugated estrogen (0.625 PO q.d.) and medroxyprogesterone (2.5 mg q.d.)

   3. **Available estrogens and starting doses**

a. Micronized estradiol (Estrace)	1 mg q.d.
b. 17-B estradiol (Estraderm patch)	0.05 mg 2×/wk
c. Esterified estergen (Estratab)	0.625 mg q.d.
d. Estropipate (Ogen)	0.625 mg q.d.
e. Conjugated estrogens (Premarin)	0.625 mg q.d.

   4. **Available progestins and starting doses**

     a. Medroxyprogesterone acetates

i. Amen	2.5–10 mg q.d.
ii. Curretab	2.5–10 mg q.d.
iii. Cycrin	2.5–10 mg q.d.
iv. Provera	2.5–10 mg q.d.

     b. Norethindrone

i. Micronor	0.35 mg q.d.
ii. Nor Q.D.	0.35 mg q.d.

     c. Norgestrel   0.075 mg q.d.

   5. **Special considerations**

     a. Low-dose norethindrone, if used in treatment regimen, may be found in progestin-only birth control pill

    b. If withdrawal bleeding is problematic, consider lowering estrogen dose from 0.625 mg to 0.3 mg q.d.; but this dose may not be effective in preventing osteoporosis

    c. The estrogen patch may be substituted for oral estrogen and is applied for 3 wk of every 4-wk cycle; progestin (5–10 mg) is given concurrently for 12–14 d per cycle

    d. Patients with mild hepatic dysfunction may use estrogen patch rather than oral estrogen, with LFTs monitored periodically

    e. Women who have a history of breast cancer should consult specialists before starting any type of hormone replacement therapies

IV. Monitoring

A. Women on estrogens should be seen annually for
1. Breast and pelvic examination
2. Blood pressure measurements
3. Mammography as indicated by age and risk factors
   - See chapter on "Breast Lesions" for details
4. Discussion of continuing treatment

B. If bleeding other than withdrawal bleeding occurs, refer patient to gynecologist for evaluation of endometrium

C. Women on estrogen-only therapy with intact endometrial tissue should be followed by a gynecologist

V. Referrals to Gynecologist and/or Specialist for

A. Uncertainty of treatment regimens

B. Abnormality on pelvic examination

C. Evaluation of abnormal vaginal bleeding prior to or during hormonal replacement therapy

D. Poor response to low-dose therapies above or if patient requests estrogen only replacement therapy

References

1. American College of Obstetrics and Gynecology: Estrogen replacement therapy. ACOG Tech Bull No. 93, June 1986.
2. Booher DL: Estrogen supplements in menopause. Cleve Clin J Med 57:154–160, 1990.
3. Notelovitz M: Estrogen replacement therapy: Indications, contraindications, and agent selection. Am J Obstet Gynecol 161 (Part 2):1832–1841, 1989

Human Immunodeficiency Virus: General Approach

I. Definition

A. The human immunodeficiency viruses (HIV-1 and -2)

1. Are cytopathic retroviruses of the lentivirus group
2. Are transmitted by direct contact with infected secretions and blood products
3. Infect human T lymphocytes, CD4 (helper) type, as well as other cell lines
4. Cause acquired immunodeficiency syndrome (AIDS)

II. General Principles

A. Physicians are ethically and morally responsible for treating HIV-positive patients
B. The following adult individuals/groups are considered at higher risk for HIV infection
   1. Homosexual and bisexual men (especially those engaging in unprotected anal intercourse)
   2. Intravenous drug users who share needles
   3. Hemophiliacs and recipients of blood products, especially prior to June 1985
   4. Anyone with multiple sexual partners, especially with a history of previous sexually transmitted diseases
   5. Persons engaging in intimate sexual relations with the above risk groups
   6. Health-care workers with puncture injury from HIV needle or sharp instrument
C. The estimated time from initial HIV infection to
   1. Nonspecific symptoms (e.g., weight loss, fatigue): 6–8 yr
   2. AIDS: 8–12 yr
D. Estimated time from diagnosis of AIDS to death is 18–24 mo
E. CD4 counts decrease at an approximate rate of 50 counts/yr
F. The death rate when CD4 counts are above 200 is approximately 1–2%/yr
   1. From 50–200 counts the death rate is 5–15%/yr
   2. Below 50 the death rate approaches 50%/yr
G. Seroconversion usually occurs within 3 mo of infection with HIV

III. Serologic Tests

A. Enzyme-linked immunoabsorbent assay (ELISA)
   1. This method usually detects antibodies after seroconversion
   2. Screening is initially with ELISA
   3. False-positive tests may occur in low-risk asymptomatic individuals
B. Western blot test is used to confirm positive ELISA tests
C. P-24 antigen is used for staging and evaluating infectivity
D. Polymerized chain reaction (PCR) is the most sensitive way to detect HIV but is not at present routinely available

IV. Diagnostics

A. **History**
   1. Identification of risk group
   2. Probable date of onset

   3. Presence of systemic and organ-specific symptoms
      a. General: fatigue, weakness, malaise, weight loss, fever, night sweats, lymph node enlargement
      b. Skin: dry skin (xeroderma), flaky facial rash, purple lesions
      c. HEENT: visual changes, mouth pain or ulcers, dysphagia
      d. Cardiorespiratory: dyspnea, chronic cough, chest tightness
      e. GI: diarrhea, perianal pain, or ulcer
      f. GU: genital ulcers, urinary difficulties, vaginitis, vaginal or urethral discharge
      g. Extremities: peripheral pain, tingling or numbness, joint pain
      h. Neurologic: changes in personality, memory
   4. Medical history of possible complications of HIV
      a. Skin: seborrheic dermatitis, eczema, psoriasis, Kaposi's sarcoma, herpes infections
      b. STD and infectious diseases: syphilis, HSV, PID, TB, HbC, amebiasis, gonococcus
      c. Opportunistic infections: PCP, oral esophageal candidiasis, cryptococcal meningitis, toxoplasmosis, MAI, cryptosporidiosis, *M. tuberculosis*
      d. Neoplasia: lymphoma or carcinomata
      e. Neurologic: seizures or dementia
   5. Immune and vaccination status: measles, mumps, rubella, varicella, tetanus, polio, influenza, pneumococcal
   6. Medications
B. **Examination**
   1. Examination must be detailed and thorough
   2. Focus on findings of above
C. **Laboratory data**
   1. For screening use ELISA and Western Blot
   2. **Initial investigations** for HIV-infected patients
      a. CBC with a differential, platelet count
      b. Electrolytes, glucose, BUN, creatinine
      c. Liver function tests
      d. Urinalysis
      e. PPD with controls
      f. Syphilis serology (VDRL or RPR)
      g. T-lymphocyte subsets (CD4 count)
      h. Hepatitis B serology
      i. Toxoplasmosis titers
      j. Chest x-ray

V. **Management**

A. **General approach**
   1. Discuss safe sexual behavior: abstinence is the most effective method, followed by use of condoms with spermicidal lubricant

2. Discuss importance of notifying current or past sexual and/or needle partner
3. Ensure patient has up-to-date immunization status
4. Assure patient of confidentiality
5. Referrals as appropriate
   a. Mental health counseling
   b. Social worker for advice on
      i. Social and professional support groups
      ii. Housing and shelters
      iii. Disability
      iv. Obtaining medication
   c. Nutritional assessment, especially for patients with weight loss and diarrhea
6. For substance abusers, discuss referral to a rehabilitation program
7. Phone number for the AIDS Hotline: (800) 342-2437
8. Information on current clinical trials from AmFAR: (800) 874-2572

B. **Treatment protocols**
1. **Summary of staging by CD4 levels and treatment with AZT**
   a. If CD4 count is
      i. >600, repeat within 6 mo
      ii. 500–600, repeat within 3 mo
      iii. <500, repeat 1 wk later
         (a) If still <500, begin zidovudine (AZT)
            (i) 200 mg q4 for 1 mo
            (ii) 100 mg q4 thereafter
         (b) Monitor CD4 count in 3–6 mo
      iv. <300, repeat count within 3 mo and treat with AZT as above
      v. <200
         (a) Initiate PCP prophylaxis
         (b) Treat with AZT, as above
         (c) Further CD4 counts will not change management
2. **Zidovudine** (AZT)
   a. **Side effects**
      i. Nausea, headache, myopathy, anemia, and granulocytopenia
      ii. Most symptoms, except for hematological side effects, resolve after several wk
      iii. Drug interactions include increased risk of neurotoxicity when given with acyclovir
   b. **Monitoring**
      i. Clinical evaluation within 2 wk of starting AZT and at regular intervals thereafter
      ii. Obtain baseline CBC prior to beginning therapy, then monthly for 3 mo, and then every 3 mo thereafter

        iii. Other monitoring tests may include CPK and LDH every 3 mo for those patients who have been on AZT >6 mo

        iv. For patients intolerant of AZT or who significantly deteriorate while on AZT, consider use of dideoxyinosine (DDI)

3. **Dideoxyinosine** (DDI)
  a. Indications
      i. Intolerance of AZT
      ii. Significant deterioration while on AZT (including AZT-induced anemia)
  b. Dosing of DDI
      i. For patients >75 kg
          (a) Tablets: 300 mg q12
          (b) Powder form: 375 mg (in water) q12
      ii. For patients 50–74 kg
          (a) Tablet form: 200 mg q12
          (b) Powder form: 250 mg (in water) q12
  c. Special considerations
      i. Take pills on empty stomach
      ii. Chew or crush pills before ingesting
  d. Adverse reactions include pancreatitis, peripheral neuropathy (characterized by tingling, numbness), headache, and diarrhea

4. *Pneumocystis carinii* **pneumonia (PCP) prophylaxis**
  a. Should begin after known PCP pneumonia or episode of oral thrush or if CD4 count <200
  b. **Prophylaxis alternatives**
      i. **Trimethoprim/sulfamethoxazole**
          (a) Recommended regimen: 160/800 mg q.d. for life is the preferred prophylactic regimen, but it has a relatively high rate of adverse effects
          (b) Adverse effects include rash, neutropenia, interstitial nephritis, hemolysis in G6PDH deficiency
      ii. **Pentamidine**
          (a) 300 mg by aerosol q 4 wk
          (b) Adverse effects include hyperglycemia, hypoglycemia, pancreatitis
          (c) Caution should be used with
              (i) Diabetics
              (ii) Asthmatics
          (d) Pentamidine is not completely protective but should be used if patient intolerant of trimethoprim/sulfamethoxazole
          (e) Before beginning aerosol treatment patient must be assessed for *M. tuberculosis* by
              (i) Clinical evaluation
              (ii) Tuberculin test (PPD)
              (iii) CXR

        (f) If patient has cough or abnormal CXR, send at least 3 sputum samples for AFB smears and culture

        (g) Discontinue aerosol if signs of PCP infection develop

     iii. For alternative prophylactic regimens (i.e., dapsone), contact ID specialist for details

C. Opportunistic infections and other problems

1. Neurologic

a. Cryptococcal meningitis

    i. Usually presents with headache and fever without stiff neck

    ii. Laboratory studies

        (a) CSF: glucose (low), India ink stain, cryptococcal antigen

        (b) Serum cryptococcal antigen

    iii. Consult with ID specialist for details of treatment, which will consist of

        (a) Amphotericin with or without fluorocytosine

b. Progressive multifocal leukoencephalopathy (PML)

    i. Due to parvovirus

    ii. No curative treatment

c. HIV encephalopathy

    i. Cause of HIV dementia

    ii. Consider higher doses of AZT

d. Toxoplasmosis

    i. Persons with negative titers have toxoplasmosis <5% of time

    ii. Clinical toxoplasmosis is usually due to reactivated infection

    iii. If titers positive and patient asymptomatic, no treatment is required (except if patient has brain lesions due to toxoplasmosis)

    iv. With headache and fever and/or neurologic symptoms, consider CT scan of brain with contrast looking for ring-enhancing lesions

    v. Treat with pyrimethamine, sulfadiazine, and folinic acid

        (a) Consult ID specialist for details

2. Candidiasis

a. Oral thrush may be treated with any of

    i. Clotrimazole troches: 5 ×/d

    ii. Nystatin suspension: 5 ml, swish and spit or swallow, q.i.d.

    iii. Ketoconazole: 200–400 mg PO q.d. for 14 d

        (a) This drug may be less well absorbed in patients with HIV infection

    iv. Fluconazole: 100 mg PO q.d. for 14 d

   b. **Candidal esophagitis**
      i. Endoscopy may assist in differentiating thrush from other causes of esophagitis (e.g., HSV, CMV)
      ii. Drug regimens include one of
         (a) Ketoconazole: 200–400 mg PO q.d. 14–21 d
         (b) Fluconazole: given as a first dose of 200 mg, then 100 mg q.d. for 14–21 d
      iii. Ketoconazole is not well absorbed with H_2-blockers or omeprazole
      iv. Ketoconazole should not be given concurrently with terfenadine or astemizole
      v. **Note:** there is no consensus on duration of therapy; consult with GI or ID specialist for recommended regimen
      vi. May need to admit for IV amphotericin if candidiasis does not respond to oral therapy
         • See chapter on "HIV and GI Infections" for further details
3. **Herpes simplex:** for severe mucocutaneous disease
   a. Acyclovir: 200 mg PO, 5×/d for 10 d
   b. Consider IV acyclovir
   c. Patient may need suppressive therapy
      • See chapter on "STDs" for details
4. **Herpes varicella-zoster**
   a. For dermatomal zoster, consider use of acyclovir: 800 mg PO 5×/d for 7–10 d
   b. For disseminated HVZ, consider IV acyclovir
5. **Cytomegalovirus retinitis**
   a. Refer to ophthalmologist for assessment and/or documentation of retinitis
   b. Treat with IV ganciclovir or foscarnet
   c. Consult ID specialist for details
6. **For disseminated *Mycobacterium avium-intracellulare***
   a. This is often not treated
   b. Treatment regimens should be discussed with an ID specialist and may include combination therapy with
      i. Rifampin: 600 mg PO q.d.
      ii. Ethambutol: 15–25 mg/kg PO q.d.
      iii. Clofazimine: 100–300 mg PO q.d.
      iv. Ciprofloxacin: 750 mg PO q.d.
   c. Other drugs may include
      i. Amikacin: 7.5 mg/kg IV or IM q.d.
      ii. Clarithromycin: 500–1000 mg PO q.d.
      iii. Azithromycin: 600–1200 mg q.d.
7. **Tuberculosis or PPD-positivity**
   • See chapter on "HIV and Tuberculosis" for details
8. **Syphilis**
   • See chapter on "HIV and Syphilis" for details

9. **GI infections and diarrhea**
   - See chapter on "HIV and GI Infections" for details
10. **Kaposi sarcoma**
    - For severe disease refer to oncologist or ID specialist
11. **Anemia**
    a. Evaluate for vitamin deficiencies and/or GI bleeding
    b. If patient on AZT and anemia has no other treatable cause and serum erythropoietin level <500 IU
       i. Consider erythropoietin therapy
       ii. Consult hematologist for details
    c. If anemia considered secondary to AZT therapy, consider substituting DDI for AZT

VI. **Referral to an ID Specialist for**
   A. Uncertainty of management
   B. Treatment of opportunistic infections
   C. Complicated HIV or AIDS cases

References

1. Centers for Disease Control: Recommendations for prophylaxis against *Pneumocystis carinii* pneumonia for adults and adolescents infected with human immunodeficiency virus. MMWR 41 (RR-4), April, 1992.
2. Drugs for AIDS and associated infections. Med Lett 33:95–102, 1991.
3. Harrison's Principles of Internal Medicine, 12th ed. New York, McGraw-Hill, 1991.
4. HIV Early Care: AMA Physician Guidelines. Chicago, American Medical Association, 1991.
5. Volberding PA, Lagakos SW, Koch MA, et al: Zidovudine in asymptomatic human immunodeficiency virus infection: A controlled trial in persons with fewer than 500 CD4-positive cells per cubic millimeter. N Engl J Med 322:941–949, 1990.

Human Immunodeficiency Virus: GI Infections

I. **General Principles**
   A. GI problems affect 30–50% of persons with AIDS in U.S.
   B. Diarrhea may be a temporary occurrence at time of seroconversion
   C. Diarrhea in AIDS is often characterized by
      1. Large-volume stools with blood
      2. Abdominal pain
      3. Greater degrees of immunosuppression (lower CD4 counts) than in persons without diarrhea
      4. Greater weight loss than in those without diarrhea
   D. Esophageal disease is frequent among persons with AIDS
      1. Candidal esophagitis is most common
      2. Other etiologies include

      a. CMV and HSV
      b. Mycobacterium *(M TB, MAI)*
      c. Other fungi such as *Histoplasma capsulatum*
      d. Neoplasms such as Kaposi's sarcoma
      e. Idiopathic causes
      f. Multiple causes (in up to 50% of patients)

E. **Common opportunistic organisms** and sites of infection

1.	*Candida albicans*	Esophagus
2.	*Isospora belli*	Small intestine
3.	*Salmonella* species	Small intestine
4.	*Giardia*	Small intestine
5.	*Microsporidium*	Small intestine
6.	*Myco. avium-intracellulare*	Stomach to colon
7.	*Cryptosporidium* species	Small and large intestine
8.	*Campylobacter*	Small and large intestine
9.	*Clostridium difficile*	Colon
10.	*Histoplasma*	Colon
11.	*Shigella flexneri*	Colon
12.	*E. histolyticum*	Colon
13.	Cytomegalovirus	Anywhere in GI tract
14.	Herpes species	Esophagus, rectum

II. **Diagnostics for Diarrhea**

  A. **History**
    1. Duration of problem
    2. Characterization of diarrhea
    3. Systemic symptoms of weight loss, fevers, sweats
    4. Travel or geographic location
    5. History of infections in partner(s)
    6. Sexual practices
    7. Exposure to certain foodstuffs
    8. Medications

  B. **Examination**
    1. Vital signs for orthostasis
    2. Skin turgor
    3. Other signs of dehydration
    4. Abdominal examination
    5. Rectal examination and stool hemoccult test

  C. **Laboratory data**
    1. Stool for
      a. Smear for fecal leukocytes (can use methylene blue)
      b. Culture × 3
        i. Salmonella
        ii. Shigella
      c. Assay *C. difficile* toxin
    2. Stool specimens (direct, concentrated, or both) × 3
      a. For ova and parasites using various preparations
        i. Saline
        ii. Iodine

        iii. Acid-fast stain
        iv. Trichrome
   3. If clinical evaluation suggests dehydration
     a. Electrolytes, creatinine, BUN

III. Management of Diarrhea

A. General approach

1. It is best **not** to treat empirically (because potential pathogens are too numerous) unless patient is very toxic or has fecal leakage
   a. Consult ID for suggested regimen
2. Give fluids, oral electrolytes (e.g., Gatorade or equivalent), if needed
3. If bacterial infection is suspected, avoid antidiarrheal therapy

B. If initial investigations do not identify pathogens

1. Refer to GI for further diagnostic tests
   a. Gastroscopy
   b. Duodenoscopy
   c. Colonoscopy with biopsies and fluid specimens

C. If specific pathogen identified, give PO medications

1. For *Salmonella* species
   a. Amoxicillin: 1 g t.i.d. for 3–14 d
   b. Trim/sulfa: 160/800 mg b.i.d. for 14 d
   c. Ciprofloxacin: 500 mg b.i.d. for 1 wk
2. For *Shigella* species
   a. Trim/sulfa: 160/800 mg b.i.d. for 5–15 d
   b. Ciprofloxacin: 500 mg b.i.d. for 1 wk
   c. Ampicillin: 500 mg q.i.d. for 5 d
3. For *Campylobacter*
   a. Erythromycin: 250–500 mg q.i.d. for 1 wk
   b. Ciprofloxacin: 500 mg b.i.d. for 1 wk
4. For *C. difficile*
   a. Metronidazole: 500 mg t.i.d. for 7–10 d or 250 mg q.i.d. for 7–10 d
   b. Vancomycin: 125 mg q.i.d. for 7–10 d
5. For *Giardia lamblia*
   a. Metronidazole: 250 mg t.i.d. for 5 d
   b. Quinacrine: 100 mg t.i.d. for 5 d

IV. Diagnostics for Esophageal Pain or Dysphagia

A. History

1. Presence of dysphagia and/or pain on swallowing and severity of symptoms
2. Ability to tolerate fluids and foods
3. Anorexia and weight loss
4. GI bleeding, melena
5. Medications such as NSAIDs

B. Examination

1. Oral examination for ulcerations, candidiasis
2. Neck examination for masses, lymphadenopathy
3. Abdominal palpation for masses, epigastric tenderness
4. Fecal occult blood test

C. **Laboratory data**
   1. Initial investigations may not be necessary
   2. **Further investigations**
      a. **Barium swallow**
         i. Frequently used in evaluation of esophageal symptoms, particularly dysphagia
            (a) Candidal esophagitis may be seen as: numerous plaque-like lesions or nodular lesions (infrequently)
            (b) HSV disease may be seen as multiple ulcerations, usually <1.5 mm in diameter
            (c) CMV esophagitis may be seen as large, single or multiple ulcerations
         ii. Barium studies may not be accurate in picking up mild or early candidal disease and usually cannot indicate when esophageal disease has >1 cause
      b. **Endoscopy**
         i. Allows visualization and biopsy of lesions, when present
         ii. Preferred method of diagnosing esophageal problems in HIV-infected persons

V. **Management of Esophageal Disease**

A. **General approach**
   1. For esophagitis presumed secondary to medications
      a. Discontinue drug causing symptoms
      b. If no improvement in symptoms, consider endoscopic evaluation
   2. For GI reflux symptoms
      a. Consider trial of therapy of 7–10 d with H_2-antagonist of choice
         • See chapter on "Dyspepsia" for details
      b. If no improvement in symptoms, consider endoscopic evaluation
      c. If symptoms improve, consider 6–8 wk course of H_2-blocker
   3. For mild esophageal pain or dysphagia
      a. Consider a trial of therapy with an antifungal drug (see below) for 7–10 d
      b. If no improvement in symptoms, consider endoscopic evaluation
      c. If symptoms improve, consider full course of ketoconazole or fluconazole or equivalent antifungal therapy
         i. **Note:** There is no consensus on duration of therapy

4. For severe symptoms (e.g., decreased fluid and/or food intake, weight loss, melena or hemoccult-positive stool), refer for endoscopy

B. **Pharmacologic treatment**
   1. For candidal esophagitis, consider either of
      a. Ketoconazole: 200–400 mg/d, up to 8 wk (usually 2–3 wk)
      b. Fluconazole: 100 mg/d, up to 8 wk (usually 2–3 wk)
   2. For HSV esophagitis
      a. Acyclovir: PO 200–400 mg 5×/d
         or
      b. Admit for IV therapy
   3. For CMV or histoplasmosis, admit for specific IV therapies

VI. **Referral to a Gastroenterologist or ID Specialist for**

A. Uncertainty of diagnosis or management
B. Failure to diagnose cause of diarrhea
C. For severe esophageal disease
D. Failure of medical treatment of GI problem
E. Recurrent infection or symptoms
F. For treatment options for pathogens not described above

References

1. NIH Conference: Gastrointestinal infections in AIDS. Ann Intern Med 116:63–77, 1992.
2. Wilcox CM: Esophageal disease in the acquired immunodeficiency syndrome: Etiology, diagnosis, and management. Am J Med 92:412–421, 1992.

Human Immunodeficiency Virus: Syphilis

I. **General Principles**

A. Serologic response to *T. pallidum* is usually normal in HIV patients
B. HIV patients infected by sexual contact or through IV drug abuse should be tested for syphilis
C. Persons with syphilis should be advised to be tested for HIV
D. Classification of syphilis stages
   1. **Early syphilis**
      a. Primary or secondary disease
      b. Early latent disease
   2. **Late syphilis**
      a. Duration >1 yr
      b. Cardiovascular syphilis
      c. Gummas
      d. Late latent disease

     3. **Neurosyphilis:** spinal fluid may have any of
       a. Total protein >40 mg/100 ml or
       b. Cell count >5 mm^3
       c. VDRL may be positive or negative

II. Diagnostics

A. History
1. Presumed infection date
2. Sexual behavior (number of partners, type of sexual practice)
3. Presence of chancre or rash
4. Fevers
5. Previous syphilis tests and/or treatment
6. Neurologic symptoms

B. Examination
1. Search for oral, genital, anorectal chancres
2. Lymphadenopathy
3. Rash
4. Neurological evaluation

C. Laboratory data
1. Initial screening is by VDRL test (or RPR)
    a. Considered positive if dilution is 1:8
    b. May be positive if dilution is 1:4
2. If serology is positive, then CSF should be examined if
    a. Any neurological abnormalities exist
    b. Previous treatment fails
    c. Patient has had syphilis >1 yr or of unknown duration
    d. Patient has not had penicillin treatment

III. Management

A. If clinical evaluation is normal and screening test positive
1. Treat as early disease
2. If present >1 yr or duration unknown
    a. CSF examination for neurosyphilis
       i. If positive, treat with regimen below
       ii. If negative, treat as late latent syphilis
       iii. If patient refuses LP, treat as neurosyphilis
B. If clinical evaluation suggests syphilis but screening is not positive
1. Request further tests (DFA-TP, FTA-ABS, MHA-TP, dark-field microscopy, or tissue biopsy)
2. Consult with or refer to ID specialist or STD clinic

IV. Treatment

A. For early syphilis (<1 yr duration)
1. Benzathine PCN G: 2.4 mU IM, 1 dose
    a. This regimen may not be efficacious in persons who are HIV-infected

        i. Some authorities recommend the above dose, given q wk × 3 wk, as in treating late disease

       ii. Consult with ID specialist for latest information

  2. For PCN-allergic patients, either of

    a. Doxycycline: 100 mg b.i.d. × 14 d

    b. Tetracycline: 500 mg q.i.d. × 14 d

B. For late syphilis

  1. Benzathine PCN G: 2.4 mU IM, q wk for 3 wk

  2. For PCN-allergic patients

    a. Doxycycline: 100 mg b.i.d. × 30 d

    b. Tetracycline: 500 mg q.i.d. × 30 d

C. For neurosyphilis (outpatient regimen)

  1. Aqueous procaine PCN G: 2.4 mU IM q.d. × 10–14 d and

  2. Probenecid: 500 mg q.i.d. × 10–14 d

    a. Probenecid is contraindicated in patients receiving AZT therapy

  3. **Note:** there is concern that this is not effective in HIV-infected persons and that treatment should be discussed with an ID specialist

  4. Patients who are symptomatic with neurologic dysfunction and/or altered mental status should be hospitalized

V. Monitoring for HIV-Infected Patients

A. Repeat titer at 1, 2, 3 mo and 3 mo thereafter until serologic response seen

  1. For primary syphilis, >2 dilution decrease at 3 mo

  2. For secondary syphilis, same by 6 mo

  3. If response fails to occur or titer rises twofold, reassess by screening tests and CSF examination

B. **Sexual partners**

  1. Advise patient to have partner(s) evaluated and considered for treatment

C. **Notification**

  1. Notify state agency for social worker follow-up

VI. Referral to ID Specialist or STD Clinic for

A. Uncertainty of diagnosis or treatment

B. Further evaluation of patient who has no response or minimal response to treatment

C. Suspected syphilis in a patient with negative screening tests

D. Neurosyphilis

References

1. Centers for Disease Control: Recommendations for diagnosing and testing syphilis in HIV-infected patients. MMWR 37:601–608, 1988.
2. CDC Guidelines for Treatment of STD. 38(S-8):5–15, 1989.

Human Immunodeficiency Virus: Tuberculosis

I. General Principles

A. Incidence of TB in AIDS patients is 500× the incidence in the general population
   1. A negative PPD does not exclude the diagnosis
   2. Blacks and Hispanics 25–44 y/o have a particularly high incidence
   3. The prevalence of active TB in HIV-infected patients is estimated at 8%/yr
   4. Pulmonary TB is not an AIDS-defining illness, though extrapulmonary disease is. Extrapulmonary TB
      a. Occurs in 24–45% of patients with HIV-infection
      b. Occurs in up to 70% of patients with TB and AIDS

B. HIV-infected individuals have poor delayed hypersensitivity response and hence less induration from a positive PPD

II. Diagnostics

A. History and examination
   1. Specific symptoms may include
      a. Weight loss and fevers
      b. Temperatures >39.5° C
      c. Lymphadenopathy and lymphadenitis
      d. GU or GI complaints
      e. Headaches and/or meningoencephalitic symptoms
   • See chapter on "Tuberculosis" for futher details

B. Laboratory data
   1. The routine evaluation for HIV-infected persons includes
      a. PPD
         i. Some practitioners recommend 2 controls be placed as well
         ii. A positive PPD in an HIV-infected person is 5 mm or more of induration
         iii. If PPD is positive, evaluate CXR for signs of TB
            (a) Hilar adenopathy–42%
            (b) Pleural effusions–29%
            (c) Upper lobe infiltrates–25%
            (d) Miliary pattern–13%
            (e) Cavitation–6%
      b. CXR
         i. May have abnormalities consistent with TB but without a concomitant positive PPD
         ii. TB often has atypical pattern in HIV-infected persons
   2. If CXR indicates possible TB, send 3 sputum for acid-fast smear and TB cultures

a. 31–82% have positive acid-fast smears of sputum
b. Delayed diagnosis is often due to too few sputum samples analyzed
c. Consider inducing sputum, when necessary, with aero-solized hypertonic saline

3. In some patients consider
   a. Urinalysis for sterile pyuria
   b. Bronchoscopy with washings and biopsy may be necessary for further evaluation if sputum are nondiagnostic
      i. 30–73% have positive AFB in bronchoalveolar-lavage fluid or in transbronchial-biopsy specimens
   c. Blood cultures have up to a 40% in extrapulmonary TB
   d. Fine needle aspiration of lymph node if lymphadenitis present
   e. Bone marrow biopsy with cultures and stains for TB
   f. Stool specimens, because AFB can sometimes be found in stool
   g. CT scan of brain if neurologic abnormalities found
      i. Ring-enhancing or hypodense masses may be tuberculoma or tuberculous abscess
   h. CSF examination if CT abnormal or TB meningitis suspected

III. **Management**

A. **In asymptomatic adults with positive PPD**
   1. **Chemoprophylaxis prevents 90% of cases of TB**
      a. Isoniazid (INH) (300 mg q.d.) and pyridoxine (50 mg q.d.) for 12 mo
   2. Chemoprophylaxis is also considered for HIV-infected persons who are anergic and have any of
      a. A documented history of positive PPD in without treatment
      b. CXR abnormalities suggestive of previous untreated tuberculosis
      c. Close contact with TB-infected individuals
      d. Consult with ID specialist, prior to beginning prophylaxis for these persons

B. **In a patient with a positive PPD and evidence of pulmonary TB**
   1. **General approach**
      a. Optimal therapy for HIV-infected and AIDS persons is still unknown
      b. Long-term therapy is based on culture and sensitivity results
   2. **Initial therapy**
      a. If no drug resistance suspected
         i. Isoniazid, rifampin, pyrazinamide
      b. If drug resistance possible
         i. Isoniazid, rifampin, pyrazinamide, ethambutol

3. **Long-term therapy**
    a. Drug-susceptible organisms are treated with isoniazid, rifampin, and pyrazinamide for 2 mo, then isoniazid and rifampin for 7 mo or 6 mo after cultures are negative (whichever is longer)
    b. Isoniazid-resistant organisms are treated with rifampin and ethambutol for 18 mo or for 12 mo after cultures are negative (whichever is longer)
        i. Pyrazinamide is occasionally used
    c. Patients intolerant of rifampin are treated with isoniazid, pyrazinamide, and ethambutol for 18–24 mo or 12 mo after cultures are negative (whichever is longer)
        i. Pyridoxine is frequently given with INH
    d. **Dosages**
        i. Rifampin: 600 mg q.d., with reduced dose to 450 mg if weight <50 kg
        ii. Isoniazid: 300 mg q.d.
        iii. Pyrazinamide: 25 mg/kg/d, maximum dose 2.0 g q.d.
        iv. Ethambutol: 25 mg/kg/d, maximum dose 2.5 g q.d.
        v. Pyridoxine: 50 mg q.d.
    e. **Monitoring**
        i. Sputum samples are cultured until negative
        ii. LFTs should be monitored in initial phase of treatment with isoniazid
    f. **Adverse effects**
        • See chapter on "Tuberculosis" for details of adverse effects
    g. **Drug interactions**
        i. Ketoconazole inhibits the absorption of rifampin
        ii. Ketoconazole and fluconazole show reduced serum levels when given with rifampin and isoniazid
    h. **Infectious control**
        i. Isolation of the HIV-infected person with active TB is crucial to prevent spread of the infection, especially among other HIV-infected patients

IV. **Referral to Infectious Disease and/or Pulmonary Specialist for**
    A. Uncertainty of diagnosis or treatment
    B. Extrapulmonary TB
    C. Suspected or documented *Mycobacterium avium-intracellulare*
    D. Failure to diagnose suspected TB with PPD, CXR, and/or sputum
    E. Monitoring of treatment regimen

References

1. American Thoracic Society: Treatment of tuberculosis and tuberculosis infection in adults and children. Am Rev Respir Dis 134:355–362, 1986.

2. Barnes et al: Tuberculosis in patients with human immunodeficiency virus infection. N Engl J Med 324:1644–1650, 1991.
3. Centers for Disease Control: The use of preventative therapy for tuberculosis infection in the United States. MMWR May 18, 1990.
4. Centers for Disease Control: Screening for tuberculosis and tuberculosis infection in high risk populations. MMWR April 26, 1991.

Hypertension: Essential

I. Definition

Hypertension is defined as an elevation of systolic blood pressure >140 mmHg and/or diastolic blood pressure >90 mmHg

II. General Principles

A. Hypertension is the leading reason for patient visits and prescriptions in the U.S.

B. 95% of hypertension is idiopathic

C. For given levels of high blood pressures, morbidity and mortality are higher for
1. Men
2. Blacks
3. Persons with evidence of target-organ damage
4. Persons with other major coronary risk factors

D. Antihypertensive therapy reduces the incidence of CVAs, CHF, and, possibly, myocardial infarctions

E. Classification and risk categories are broken down by diastolic or systolic. Elevation of either of these above 140/90 mmHg incurs a higher risk of coronary heart disease

F. **Summary of levels of hypertension and recommended monitoring**
1. **Diastolic** (DBP) (in mmHg)
   a. <85: recommend follow-up within 2 yr
   b. 85–89 is high normal: recheck within 1 yr
   c. 90–104 is mild hypertension: recheck within 2 mo
   d. 105–114 is moderate: recheck within 2 wk
   e. Above 115 is severe: evaluate and treat within 2 d
2. **Systolic** (SBP) when **DBP** <**90** (in mmHg)
   a. 140–159 is borderline isolated systolic hypertension (ISH); recheck within 2 mo
   b. ≥160 is ISH; recheck within 2 mo
   c. >200 is severe; evaluate and treat within 2 wk
3. **Recommended methods for diagnosing hypertension**
   a. **Hypertension is diagnosed by at least 2 separate readings during 2 or 3 separate clinic appointments**
   b. Blood pressures decrease with repeated measurement
   c. Support arm while measuring pressure

   d. Measure pressures in both arms and monitor by using arm with initial higher value
   e. Diastolic reading is at disappearance of sounds (phase 5)
   f. **Record cuff size,** if large cuff used

III. **Diagnostics**

A. **History**
1. Previous diagnosis/treatment for hypertension
2. Family history: hypertension, renal disease, CHD
3. Assessment of other cardiovascular risks
   a. Definite coronary artery disease evidenced by prior MI and/or angina pectoris
   b. Family history of MI before age 55 y/o
   c. Diabetes mellitus
   d. Cigarette smoking >10/d, currently
   e. Cerebrovascular or peripheral vascular disease
   f. >30% overweight
   g. HDL <35 mg/dl
4. Renal disease
5. Headaches, blurry vision
6. Medications and drug use (e.g., cocaine, amphetamines)

B. **Examination**
1. General
   a. BP in both arms (use higher for monitoring)
   b. Neck examination for goiter
   c. Palpation of peripheral pulses
   d. Auscultation for bruits: carotids, femoral, renal, abdominal
   e. Abdominal exam for masses (AAA, renal mass)
2. Specific evaluation for acute or chronic target organ damage
   a. Retinopathy: arteriolar narrowing, hemorrhages, exudates
   b. LVH: S4, LV heave
   c. CHF: JVD, S3, peripheral edema
   d. Previous CVA or old focal neurologic signs
   e. Bruits (carotid, abdominal, flank, femoral)
   f. Diminished or absent peripheral pulses

C. **Laboratory data**
1. **Routine**
   a. CBC
   b. Urinalysis
   c. Creatinine and BUN
   d. Serum K, Na, glucose, and calcium
   e. Nonfasting cholesterol
   f. Electrocardiogram
2. **For selected patients**
   a. Liver function tests
   b. Serum uric acid if diuretic treatment planned
   c. Ambulatory BP monitoring

      i. Not usually cost-effective but indications include
  - (a) Suspected extreme BP lability
  - (b) Diagnosis of white-coat hypertension

      ii. Home or workplace measurements may also be used to establish trends in BP

d. Echocardiography
  - i. Indications
    - (a) Suspected cardiac abnormality
      - (i) Valvular disease
      - (ii) Cardiac failure
      - (iii) Previous myocardial infarct
    - (b) Evaluation of ventricular hypertrophy
      - (i) If EKG is nondiagnostic
      - (ii) When knowledge of hypertrophy will change management or drug choice

e. Urine drug tests for suspected cocaine or amphetamine abuse

IV. Management

A. General approach

1. If chronic target organ damage is found or laboratory result points to such (e.g., LVH), complete clinical and laboratory evaluations and start drug treatment
2. Blood pressures should be reduced gradually to minimize risk of potential complications from rapidly decreasing cerebral blood flow
3. General goals of therapy
   a. Reduce BP below 140/90
   b. For ISH, reduce BP to below 160 mmHg
   c. **Note:** For ISH of 160–179 mmHg, goal is reduction by at least 20 mmHg
4. In patients with mild HTN, without target organ damage, initial treatment is nonpharmacologic therapy; if this fails to control pressure over 3–6 mo, begin drug therapy
5. Some practitioners prefer to monitor and give only non-pharmacologic advice to asymptomatic persons with DBP <95 mmHg when they have no other CHD risk factors or target organ damage

B. Guidelines for raised **diastolic BP**

1. **If DBP is 85–89 mmHg (high-normal)**
   a. Monitor again within 1 yr
   b. Give advice on nonpharmacologic treatment (see below)
2. **If DBP is <105 mmHg (mild)**
   a. Monitor again twice over 3–4 mo before initiating therapy, unless there is evidence of nonacute target organ damage
   b. Give advice on nonpharmacologic treatment (see below)
   c. **If there is any target organ damage**
      i. Begin clinical and laboratory evaluation and start drug therapy

ii. See again within 2 wk
3. **If DBP is 105–114 mmHg (moderate)**
   a. If evidence of target organ damage, evaluate and begin treatment immediately
   b. If no target organ damage, monitor again within 2 wk
   c. If DBP still elevated after 2 wk, begin laboratory evaluation and start drug therapy
4. **If DBP is 115–140 mmHg (severe)**
   a. Begin laboratory evaluation immediately
   b. Start drug therapy
5. **If DBP is >140 (urgent)**
   • See chapter on "Hypertension: Urgent and Emergent"
6. **If acute target organ damage is found at any BP, admit for IV antihypertensive management**

C. Guidelines for raised **systolic BP**
   1. **For borderline ISH (140–159 mmHg)**
      a. Monitor within 1 yr
      b. Give advice on nonpharmacologic treatment
   2. **For ISH 160–200 mmHg**
      a. Evaluation as for elevated DBP
      b. Initial treatment is nonpharmacologic
      c. If nonpharmacologic treatment fails, start drug therapy
      d. Treatment is indicated in all age groups
   3. **For ISH >200 mmHg**
      a. Managed as for moderate (105–114 mmHg) DBP elevation, outlined above

D. **Nonpharmacologic advice**
   1. **Weight reduction** to within 15% of recommended weight
   2. **Reduce salt intake** (4–6 g/d)
      a. Especially in elderly and in African-Americans
      b. Can use salt substitute such as KCl
      c. Warn about high salt content in prepackaged foods
   3. **Decrease alcohol** to less than 2 drinks (2 oz)/d
   4. **Aerobic exercise** (e.g., walking, fitness classes, swimming) for 20–30 min at least 3 ×/wk
   5. **Relaxation** therapies such as yoga or biofeedback may be helpful
   6. **Reduce other cardiac risk factors**
      a. Stop smoking
      b. Monitor cholesterol levels
      c. Reduce saturated fats
         i. Polyunsaturated fats may help reduce BP
   7. Give **educational materials** on risks and treatment goals of hypertension

E. **Pharmacologic therapy**
   1. Avoid polypharmacy or combination drugs whenever possible
   2. **First-line drugs** (for specifics see below)
      a. Diuretics (in low doses)

    b. Beta-adrenergic blockers

    c. Calcium channel antagonists

    d. Angiotensin-converting enzyme (ACE) inhibitors

3. **If control not achieved with single first-line drug**

    a. **Increase first drug** (this is preferred method) **or**

    b. Substitute a new drug **or**

    c. Add new drug

4. Continue process until good control is achieved

5. If control not achieved by addition of third drug, ensure that patient is compliant with regimen and, if so, consider investigating secondary causes of hypertension (see next chapter for details)

V. **Drug Selection (Selected List)**

A. **Diuretics**

Drug	Maintenance Dose	Maximum Dosage
Chlorthalidone	12.5–25 mg q.d.	50 mg/d
Chlorothiazide	25–50 mg q.d.	100 mg/d
Hydrochlorothiazide (HCTZ)	12.5–25 mg q.d.	50 mg/d
Indapamide	2.5 mg q.d.	5 mg/d
Trichloromethazide	1–2 mg q.d.	4 mg/d
Triamterene	50–100 mg b.i.d.	100 mg/d
Spironolactone	25–100 mg q.d.	100 mg/d

1. Monitor electrolytes (particularly K), creatine, and BUN

2. **Adverse effects**

    a. Hypokalemia with thiazide and sulfonamide diuretics

        i. Indications for K supplementation with diuretics

            (a) Serum K is initially <3 mEq/L

            (b) Patient becomes hypokalemic

            (c) Symptoms of hypokalemia develop

            (d) When CHF is being treated

            (e) Digitalis given concurrently

        ii. Some practitioners prefer to use a potassium-sparing diuretic in addition to a thiazide diuretic to reduce potassium wasting

    b. Using a high dose of a diuretic (i.e., HCTZ to 50 mg q.d.) does not often increase effectiveness but may increase risk of side effects (e.g., hypokalemia)

    c. Thiazide diuretics may worsen glucose intolerance and hyperuricemia and raise lithium and triglyceride levels

    d. Potassium-sparing diuretics may cause hyperkalemia

        i. Especially in those who are elderly, diabetic, or who have renal insufficiency

        ii. Risk increases when these drugs (alone or combined with a thiazide as in Maxzide or Dyazide) are used with ACE inhibitors

B. **Beta-adrenergic blockers**

Drug	Maintenance Dose	Maximum Dosage
Atenolol	25–50 mg q.d.	100 mg/d
Metoprolol	50–100 mg q.d.–b.i.d.	200 mg/d
Propranolol HCL	40–60 mg b.i.d.	320 mg/d
Propranolol LA	80–160 mg q.d.	320 mg/d
Naldolol	40 mg q.d.	320 mg/d
Labetolol	100–200 mg b.i.d.	400 mg q.i.d.

1. **Adverse effects**
   a. Possible worsening of bronchospasm or CHF
   b. Fatigue, impotence, depression
   c. Decrease in HDL levels
   d. Conduction disturbances when given with calcium channel blockers

C. **ACE inhibitors**

Drug	Maintenance Dose	Maximum Dosage
Benazepril	10–40 mg q.d.–b.i.d.	80 mg/d
Captopril	12.5–50 mg b.i.d	450 mg/d
Enalapril	5–40 mg q.d.	40 mg/d
Lisinopril	5–40 mg q.d.	80 mg/d
Fosinopril	10–40 mg q.d.–b.i.d.	80 mg/d
Quinapril	10–80 mg q.d.	80 mg/d
Ramipril	2.5–10 mg q.d.–b.i.d.	20 mg/d

1. Monitor Cr, U/A (protein), K, CBC for all ACE inhibitors
2. **Adverse effects**
   a. Renal insufficiency in patients with renal artery stenosis
   b. Nonproductive cough, rashes
   c. Proteinuria
   d. Hypotension (especially when patient is dry)
   e. Hyperkalemia may occur in patients with renal insufficiency or diabetes and in patients using potassium-sparing diuretics or potassium supplementation
   f. ACE inhibitors are contraindicated in pregnancy
   g. Angioedema, rashes

D. **Calcium channel blockers**

Drug	Maintenance Dose	Maximum Dosage
Verapamil SR	120–240 mg q.d.	480 mg/d
Nifedipine XL	30–90 mg q.d.	120 mg/d
Diltiazem SR	60–120 mg b.i.d.	360 mg/d
Diltiazem CD	180–300 mg q.d.	300 mg/d
Nicardipine	20–40 mg t.i.d.	120 mg/d

1. **Adverse effects**
   a. Constipation, impotence
   b. Conduction block (drugs that slow conduction, e.g., diltiazem, are contraindicated with sick sinus syndrome and 2nd and 3rd degree heart block)
   c. Lower-extremity edema (especially nifedipine)

E. **Centrally acting**

Drug	Maintenance Dose	Maximum Dosage
Clonidine	0.1–0.6 mg b.i.d.	2.4/d
Clonidine TTS	0.1–0.3 mg patch q.wk	0.3/wk
Methyldopa	250–500 mg b.i.d.	500 q.i.d.

1. **Adverse effects**
   a. Drowsiness, sedation, fatigue
   b. Sexual dysfunction
   c. Withdrawal hypertension
   d. Coombs' positive anemia (methyldopa)

F. **Vasodilators**

Drug	Maintenance Dose	Maximum Dosage
Prazosin	1–6 mg b.i.d.	20 mg/d
Hydralazine	10–50 mg q.i.d	300 mg/d
Minoxidil	2.5–5 mg b.i.d.	100 mg/d

1. **Adverse effects**
   a. Syncope, especially prazosin, which should be started at low doses (e.g., 1 mg b.i.d.) and gradually increased so as to avoid causing syncope
   b. Reflex tachycardia
   c. Increased angina episodes
   d. Impotence
   e. Lupus-like syndrome (hydralazine)
   f. Hirsutism (minoxidil)

VI. **Special Populations**

A. **African-Americans**
   1. Respond well to diuretics and calcium channel blockers
   2. Generally do not respond as well to beta blockers or ACE inhibitors unless used with a diuretic

B. **Older patients**
   1. Benefit from treatment for elevated DBP or ISH and generally respond well to diuretics
   2. A **gradual drop** in BP is recommended

VII. **Comorbidities**

A. **LVH is an independent risk factor** for arrhythmias, sudden death
   1. Can reduce LV wall mass by weight loss and certain antihypertensives, including beta blockers, calcium antagonists, ACE inhibitors
   2. Minoxidil, hydralazine, and diuretics are not known to reduce LVH

B. **Congestive heart failure**
   1. **Diastolic dysfunction** (from LVH) with EF >40%
      a. Consider beta blockers or calcium channel blockers to increase relaxation

2. **Systolic dysfunction** with EF <40%
   a. ACE inhibitors can increase lifespan and are usually used with diuretic therapy for systolic dysfunction
C. **Peripheral vascular disease**
   1. Vascular impotence and intermittent claudication may worsen with beta blockers and may benefit from calcium antagonists, but data are not conclusive
D. **Diabetics**
   1. Beta blockers blunt hypoglycemic symptoms by interfering with catecholamine effects
   2. ACE inhibitors may aggravate hyperkalemia but may improve diabetic proteinuria
      a. Monitor serum K, Cr, BUN, urine
   3. Thiazides may worsen glucose intolerance
E. **COPD patients** may have increased bronchospasm with any beta blocker
F. **Hyperlipidemia and hypercholesteremia** may worsen with diuretics (especially thiazides) or beta blockers (cardioprotective ones may decrease HDL)
G. **Gouty arthritis** may worsen with diuretics
H. **Renal insufficiency**
   1. ACE inhibitors may lead to acute renal insufficiency (reversible) when there is bilateral renal artery stenosis
   2. Overdiuresis or overtreatment with antihypertensives may cause functional prerenal azotemia
I. **Depression** may worsen with beta blockers, clonidine, methyldopa

VIII. **Monitoring**

A. Close monitoring is needed (e.g., weekly or biweekly) while dosages are titrated upward or medications are added or changed
B. Once stable, patients should be followed periodically for
   1. Monitoring adverse effects
   2. Advice and emphasis on compliance
   3 Support for reducing other cardiac risks

IX. **Referral to Antihypertensive Specialist for**

A. Uncertainty of diagnosis and treatment
B. Failure of triple therapy to control HTN
C. If clinical evaluation or work-up suggests secondary hypertension
   • See following chapter on "Secondary Hypertension"

References

1. ACE inhibitors for hypertension. Med Lett 34:27, 1992.
2. Barker LR, Burton JR, Zieve PD: Principles of Ambulatory Care, 2nd ed. Baltimore, 1986, pp 788–828.

3. 1988 Joint National Committee: The 1988 Report of the Joint National Committee on Detection, Evaluation, and Treatment of High Blood Pressure. Arch Intern Med 148:1023–1028, 1988.
4. SHEP Cooperative Research Group: Prevention of stroke by antihypertensive drug treatment in older persons with isolated systolic hypertension. JAMA 265:3255–3264, 1991.

Hypertension: Secondary

I. **Definition**

A functional definition of secondary hypertension is an elevated systolic and/or diastolic blood pressure that can be attributed to an identifiable underlying cause

II. **General Principles**

A. Secondary hypertension is estimated to occur in less than 5% of known hypertensives
B. Causes include
   1. Renovascular hypertension with prevalence estimated at <0.5% of hypertensives
   2. Alcohol abuse
   3. Side effects of certain drugs
      a. Corticosteroids
      b. Cocaine
      c. Monoamine oxidase inhibitors
      d. Stimulants, including caffeine and nicotine
      e. Disulfiram
   4. Cushing's syndrome
   5. Primary hyperaldosteronism (Conn's syndrome)
   6. Pheochromocytoma
   7. Preeclampsia and eclampsia of pregnancy
   8. Coarctation of the aorta

III. **Diagnostics for Specific Disorders**

A. **General approach**
   1. For initial laboratory evaluation of hypertensive persons, see preceding chapter
   2. Investigation for a specific cause for hypertension should occur if
      a. Clinical evaluation suggests a cause for secondary hypertension
      b. Initial laboratory tests reveal an abnormality consistent with a cause of hypertension
      c. During medical management a secondary cause is suggested
B. **Renovascular hypertension**

1. **Indicators of possible renovascular hypertension**
   a. Severe hypertension in persons younger than 30 y/o or older than 50 y/o
   b. Sudden onset of hypertension or accelerated hypertension
   c. Significant worsening of controlled hypertension
   d. Flank or abdominal bruit (diastolic and systolic)
   e. Renal insufficiency provoked by ACE inhibitor
   f. Blood pressure >150/100 mmHg while on adequate 3 drug regimen
   g. Significant and sudden unexplained reduction in renal function in any hypertensive patient
   h. Palpable kidney
   i. Microscopic hematuria and/or proteinuria and/or active urinary sediment
   j. Widespread cardio- and/or cerebrovascular disease
2. **Laboratory data**
   a. In patients with **clinical clues** to renovascular disease, consider
      i. Renovascular scan with or without captopril administration
      ii. Plasma renin activity
      iii. Digital subtraction angiography
      iv. Renal vein sampling studies
   b. In patients who are **strongly suspected** of having renal artery stenosis (RAS), arteriography is often used as first test in conjunction with transluminal angioplasty, if lesion identified
   c. In persons with suspected renal parenchymal or obstructive disease, consider
      i. Intravenous urogram
      ii. Ultrasound of kidneys
3. **Management**
   a. **General approach**
      i. In many cases, renovascular hypertension is managed medically by single or multiple drug regimens
      ii. Reduce modifiable cardiovascular risk factors
         (a) Smoking cessation
         (b) Hyperlipidemia
         (c) Obesity
      iii. Indications for surgical intervention
         (a) Failure of medical therapy to control hypertension
         (b) Worsening renal function while on therapy
         (c) Potential for increasing renal dysfunction
            (i) Bilateral or unilateral renal artery stenosis of >75%
            (ii) Aggressively progressive lesions

iv. Patients should have **preoperative evaluation** for other cardiovascular disorders
- (a) Myocardial ischemia
- (b) Carotid disease

b. **Monitoring**
- i. Patients on medical therapy should have periodic clinical evaluation and assessment of renal function
  - (a) Cr, BUN, electrolytes
  - (b) Imaging studies such as intravenous urography or ultrasound

4. Referrals to hypertension specialist for
- a. Uncertainty of diagnosis or treatment
- b. Evaluation and management of patient with renovascular disease by above tests
- c. Failure of medical therapy for renovascular hypertension

C. **Pheochromocytoma**
1. **General approach**
- a. Characteristic **triad of symptoms** of pheochromocytoma
  - i. Sweating attacks
  - ii. Tachycardia
  - iii. Headaches
- b. Other less specific symptoms may include
  - i. Nervousness and tremor
  - ii. Facial pallor
  - iii. Nausea and occasional vomiting
  - iv. Fatigue and malaise
  - v. Weight loss
- c. Paroxysms of the above occur in about 50% of patients

2. **Pheochromocytoma should be considered in persons with**
- a. Characteristic symptoms, as above, with or without paroxysms
- b. Malignant hypertension
- c. Lack of response to adequate antihypertensive treatment
- d. Unusual or paroxysmal fluctuations of blood pressure
- e. A history of von Recklinghausen's neurofibromatosis
- f. A family history of MEN III or IIb
- g. A history of hypertension during induction of anesthesia
- h. Hypertension after starting imipramine or desipramine

3. **Diagnostics**
- a. **Clinical evaluation** should attempt to elicit symptoms and signs as noted above
  - i. Characteristic triad of symptoms, when noted in a hypertensive patient, has an accuracy of detecting pheochromocytoma with
    - (a) Sensitivity: 94%
    - (b) Specificity: 91%
  - ii. **Without characteristic triad of symptoms**
    - (a) Negative predictive value: 99.9%

    b. **Laboratory data**
       i. In patients suspected of having pheochromocytoma
         (a) Consider initial screening with a 24-hr urine collection for metanephrines, vanillylmandelic acid, or catecholamines
            (i) Negative predictive value is about 98% for any of the above tests
         (b) If screening test is positive or equivocal, confirm with second biochemical test and/or consult with an endocrinologist regarding further evaluations
  4. **Referrals** to endocrinologist or hypertension specialist for
    a. Uncertainty of diagnosis or diagnostic protocols
    b. Further evaluation after a positive or equivocal screening test(s)
    c. Suspected pheochromocytoma after negative test result(s)

D. **Cushing's syndrome**
  1. **Endogenous steroid excess** should be considered in persons with hypertension and
    a. Easy bruising
    b. Proximal myopathy
    c. Centripedal obesity and/or cushingoid appearance
    d. Red or purple striae
    e. Virilization (in women) and menstrual disturbance
    f. Hypokalemia (when noted with above symptoms)
    g. Other less specific symptoms
       i. Diabetes or glucose intolerance
       ii. Acne
  2. Excess alcohol use may produce symptoms and signs similar to Cushing's syndrome
  3. **Diagnostics**
    a. **Clinical evaluation** should attempt to elicit symptoms and signs as noted above
    b. **Laboratory data**
       i. Initial screening tests for suspected Cushing's may include either of
         (a) 24-hr urine for free cortisol
         (b) Overnight oral dexamethasone (1 mg) suppression test
            (i) Oral dose at midnight
            (ii) Plasma cortisol at 8 a.m.
       ii. In patients with positive or equivocal test results, consult with an endocrinologist for further evaluations
  4. **Referrals** to endocrinologist for
    a. Uncertainty of diagnosis or diagnostic protocol
    b. Further evaluation after a positive or equivocal screening test(s)
    c. Suspected Cushing's syndrome after negative test result(s)

References

1. Bravo EL, Gifford RW: Pheochromocytoma: Diagnosis and management. N Engl J Med 311:1298–1303, 1984.
2. Kaye TB, Crapo L: The Cushing syndrome: An update on diagnostic tests. Ann Intern Med 112:434–444, 1990.
3. Krakoff LR: Glucocortcoid excess syndromes causing hypertension. Cardiol Clin 6:537–543, 1988.
4. National Institutes of Health: Detection, evaluation, and treatment of renovascular hypertension. Arch Intern Med 147:820–829, 1987.
5. Oren S, et al: High blood pressure: Side effects of drugs, poisons, and food. Cardiol Clin 6:467–474, 1988.
6. Young MJ, et al: Biochemical tests for pheochromocytoma: Strategies in hypertensive patients. J Gen Intern Med 4:273–276, 1989.

Hypertension: Urgent and Emergent

I. **Definitions**

  A. **Urgency**
    1. DBP >140 and/or SBP >240 mmHg without complications
  B. **Emergency**
    1. **Acute end-organ damage at any BP**

II. **Diagnostics**

  A. **History of any of the following** may indicate possible acute end-organ damage
    1. Mental status changes such as behavioral change, altered sensorium
    2. Other neurological symptoms, including severe headaches, visual changes, stroke
    3. Cardiac symptoms of ischemia, aortic dissection
    4. Respiratory symptoms of dyspnea
  B. **Examination must include**
    1. Vital signs
    2. General mental status and cognition
    3. Cardiac and respiratory examination
    4. Neurologic examination
      a. Fundal assessment for
        i. Grade III: exudates and hemorrhages
        ii. Grade IV: papilledema (malignant HTN)
    5. Abdominal palpation and auscultation for bruits
  C. **Laboratory data**
    1. Urinalysis: for blood
    2. EKG: for ischemic changes
    3. CBC with smear: for anemia and hemolytic changes
    4. Electrolytes, creatinine and BUN: for renal damage

    5. CXR: for pulmonary edema, aortic dissection

    6. CT scan of head: if intracerebral or subarachnoid bleed or cerebral infarction by clinical evaluation

III. Management

A. Emergency: If acute end-organ damage found

    1. Admit for IV hypotensive medications

B. Urgency: If no acute end-organ damage found

    1. Repeat BP after getting patient relaxed and calm

    2. If BP no longer critical, refer for prompt follow-up

    3. If BP still critical, then attempt to reduce to 160–170/100 range with one of the following

       a. Nifedipine 10 mg sublingually or orally

          i. Can repeat after 30 min

         ii. Beware of precipitous drop in BP

            (a) Some physicians titrate BP, using only small amounts of nifedipine at a time

       b. Captopril 25 mg orally (can be repeated after 30 min)

       c. Prazosin 1–2 mg orally (can be repeated after 1 hr)

    4. Begin daily oral drug therapy

       • See chapter on "Hypertension" for details

    5. See patient within 48 hr

       a. To ensure response to therapy

       b. To complete evaluation

       c. To begin gradual reduction of BP to <140/90 mmHg

    6. Caution must be taken when administering acute hypertensive therapy to elderly patients and patients on concomitant antihypertensive therapy, especially diuretics (these patients may be hypovolemic)

References

1. Calhoun DA, Oparil S: Treatment of hypertensive crises. N Engl J Med 323:1177–1183, 1990.
2. Gifford RW: Management of hypertensive crises. JAMA 266:829–835, 1991.

I

Impotence

I. **Definition**

    A. Inability to obtain or sustain an erection that is satisfactory for intercourse, including

        1. Reduction in frequency of erection
        2. Lack of sufficient tumescence ("hardness") for intercourse
        3. Detumescence during intercourse

II. **General Principles**

    A. Impotence can occur at any age
    B. Coition involves stimuli in the following categories

        1. Psychogenic
        2. Vasculogenic
        3. Neurogenic
        4. Hormonal

    C. Performance anxiety often occurs with dysfunctional erection
    D. Nervous system stimuli for erection

        1. Sacral cord center: S2–S4 (reflexogenic erections)
        2. Thoracolumbar center: T12–L1 (psychogenic erections)

    E. Risk factors

        1. Increasing age
        2. Systemic diseases, especially diabetes

    F. Presence of morning and nocturnal erections strongly suggests psychogenic impotence

    G. **Causes (often multifactorial)**

        1. Psychogenic (anxiety states, stress, psychiatric distress)
        2. Anatomic
            a. Peyronie's disease = fibrous plaques in erectile bodies
        3. Endocrine
            a. Diabetes mellitus
            b. Hypogonadism
               i. Primary (testicular)
               ii. Secondary (hypothalamic–pituitary)
            c. Hyperprolactinemia
            d. Hyper- or hypothyroidism
        4. Vascular insufficiency
        5. Neuropathies
            a. Cerebrovascular
            b. Spinal
            c. Afferent
            d. Autonomic

      6. Surgery/trauma
         a. Pelvic surgery
         b. TURP
      7. Alcohol and tobacco use
      8. Medications
         a. Diuretics: HCTZ, chlorthalidone, spironolactone
         b. Antihypertensive agents: **all can cause impotence**, but particularly methyldopa, propranolol, reserpine
         c. Cimetidine
         d. Anoretic agents and anticholinergics
         e. Estrogens, antiandrogens
         f. Antidepressants and sedatives

III. **Diagnostics**

A. **History**
1. Description of erectile dysfunction
2. Age of onset
3. Presence of nocturnal and morning erections
4. History of erectile function and dysfunction
5. Psychological anxieties or other problems
6. Medications, including proprietary and prescription drugs
7. Alcohol and cigarette use
8. Symptoms of systemic disease
9. History of vascular disease and/or intermittent claudication
10. Symptoms of neurologic disease

B. **Examination**
1. Abdominal examination for masses (AAA) and bruits
2. Rectal examination of sphincter tone and prostate
3. Vascular examination for pulses and bruits
4. Signs of systemic or endocrine disease
5. Genital examination
    a. Shaft and glans of penis for anatomic lesions
    b. Testes for hypogonadism (smaller than 3.5 cm)
6. Signs of peripheral vascular disease
7. Neurologic examination for
    a. Peripheral neuropathy
    b. Perineal sensation
    c. Anal sphincter tone
    d. Vibration, position, and tactile senses

C. **Laboratory data**
1. **For selected patients when organic cause suspected**
    a. Creatinine and BUN
    b. Fasting blood sugar
    c. Urinalysis
    d. Thyroid function: TSH and FT4 or FTI
    e. Serum testosterone
    f. Serum prolactin
    g. Nocturnal penile tumescence testing is gold standard to differentiate psychogenic from organic impotence

2. **Selected tests when clinical suspicion warrants**
    a. Serum luteinizing hormone (LH): useful in differentiating secondary hypogonadism
    b. CBC and differential: if anemia suspected
3. For vasculogenic impotence
    a. Doppler ultrasound
        i. Compares penile SBP to brachial SBP
        ii. Ratio <0.7: highly suggestive of vasculogenic disorder
    b. Plethysmography measures flow across arteries of the penis and is more accurate than Doppler
    c. Papaverine testing
    d. Corpus cavernosography
4. CT scan of pituitary only if pituitary lesion is suspected by clinical or biochemical evaluation (e.g., high serum prolactin level)

IV. Management

A. General Approach
1. Psychogenic impotence may be directly referred to a psychiatrist or psychologist
2. No testing needs to be done unless organic cause is suspected
3. If medications are believed to be the cause, discontinue offending drug(s) if possible
4. Assistive devices (referral to urologist)
    a. ErecAid
        i. Pumps blood into penis by vacuum suction
        ii. Rubber constrictor prevents blood from flowing out
    b. Penile prosthesis
    c. Papaverine and other injectable vasodilators

B. For impotence due to low testosterone
1. Testosterone is treatment of choice
    a. Initial response to testosterone often tapers off over 6 mo
    b. Must ensure that patient does not have prostatic carcinoma prior to beginning testosterone therapy
        i. Digital rectal examination of prostate
        ii. Prostatic-specific antigen (PSA) levels
    c. Side effects of testosterone
        i. Gynecomastia
        ii. Rise in hematocrit
        iii. Water retention
        iv. Hypertension (secondary to water retention)
        v. Precipitation of CHF
        vi. Rapid growth of prostatic hypertrophy or cancer

C. Treatment for **neurologic impotence** may include
1. Self-injections of the corpus cavernosum with vasoactive agents
    a. Occasional priapism occurs

V. **Referral to Urologist for**
  A. Uncertainty of diagnosis or treatment
  B. Evaluation of suspected vascular impotence
  C. Further evaluation after initial tests
  D. Suspected organic cause
  E. Management of impotence not attributable to medication, endocrine, or psychogenic causes

References

1. Harrison's Principles of Internal Medicine, 12th ed. New York: McGraw-Hill, 1991, pp 296–299.
2. Maatman TJ, Montague DK, Martin ML: Cost-effective evaluation of impotence. Urology 27:132–135, 1986.
3. Morley E: Impotence. Am J Med 80:987–905, 1986.

Influenza

I. **Definition**

Influenza refers to infection with influenza viruses A or B

II. **General Principles**
  A. Vaccines for any year are developed for antigenic characteristics of that year's prominent virus strains as determined by worldwide surveillance
  B. **Vaccine** protects against **both A & B strains**
  C. **Chemoprophylaxis** (amantadine) protects **against A only**
  D. Influenza can be fatal, with **10,000–40,000 excess deaths/year**
    1. Most by pneumonia or exacerbation of cardiopulmonary disease
    2. 80–90% of deaths occur in those $\geq$ 65 y/o
  E. Vaccine is **inactivated** and is made from purified, egg-grown virus
  F. Vaccination is given any time from **September–December**
    1. Schedule depends on patient convenience and whether local area is prone to early epidemics
    2. Immunization is given yearly
  G. **Typical symptoms** of influenza
    1. Fever
    2. Sore throat
    3. Nonproductive cough
    4. Myalgia and malaise

III. **Recommendations for Immunization (Adults)**
  A. **Vaccine is recommended for high-risk patients and contacts**
    1. Persons with chronic cardiovascular and pulmonary diseases
    2. Nursing home and chronic-care facility residents

3. Those that care for the above: physicians, nurses, ancillary staff, family members
4. Persons **65 y/o or older**
5. Persons with **chronic metabolic diseases** (e.g., diabetes), **renal insufficiency** or **hemoglobinopathies**
6. Persons who are **immunosuppressed**: AIDS, posttransplant drugs
7. **Adolescents** who are on **chronic aspirin therapy** and therefore susceptible to Reye syndrome

B. Other groups
1. **Pregnant women**
    a. Especially when in high-risk group
    b. Usually after first trimester
2. Anyone who wishes to reduce risk, especially those involved with essential community services (e.g., firefighters, police)

IV. Occasional Side Effects of Vaccine

A. Soreness at injection site for 2–3 d
B. Mild fever, myalgia, and flulike symptoms for 1–2 d
C. Allergic reactions (extremely rare), mostly in persons with egg sensitivity or in persons with occupational asthma

V. Contraindication to Vaccine

A. Patients **severely allergic to egg** (i.e., hives, tongue swelling, previous anaphylaxis from eggs)

VI. Chemoprophylaxis for Influenza A Only

A. Usual adult dose: amantadine, 100 mg b.i.d.
1. Reduce for renal insufficiency
2. Reduce to 100 mg q.d. in patients > 65 y/o
B. Therapy should begin within 48 hr of abrupt onset of typical symptoms (above) or at time of exposure to virus and should be continued until 48 hr after resolution of symptoms or 10 d after exposure to virus
C. Indications for use
1. Persons who cannot tolerate immunization
    a. Give dose for as long as flu is in community
2. High-risk persons or contacts without immunization
    a. Can give for 2 wk after immunization with inactivated virus (until vaccine takes effect)
3. As an adjunct to persons with immunodeficiency
D. **Adverse reactions** (all reversible)
1. Nausea, dizziness, insomnia, agitation
2. Toxicity when renal insufficiency present
    a. Dose must be reduced
3. Increased seizure risk in those with seizure disorders
    a. Reduce dose to 100 mg q.d.

VII. **Referral**

    A. **For information on vaccine**, contact manufacturers
        1. Connaught Labs: (800) 822-2463
        2. Parke-Davis: (800) 223-0432
        3. Wyeth: (800) 321-2304

    B. **For educational materials**, contact
        1. CDC, Center for Prevention Services, Technical Information Services, 1600 Clifton Rd., NE, Atlanta, GA 30333

References

1. American Thoracic Society: Prevention of influenza and pneumonia. Am Rev Respir Dis 142:487–488, 1990.
2. Centers for Disease Control: Prevention and control of influenza: Recommendations of the Immunization Practices Advisory Committee. Ann Intern Med 107:521–525, 1987, or MMWR 36:373–387, 1987.

J

Jaundice

I. **General Principles**
   A. General classifications
      1. Hemolytic
         a. Autoimmune hemolysis
            i. Cold agglutinin disease
            ii. Drug-induced (e.g., methyldopa)
         b. Sepsis
      2. Cholestatic
         a. Hepatocellular (ETOH, hepatitis viruses)
         b. Extrahepatic
         c. Intrahepatic
   B. Initial clinical and laboratory evaluation
      1. Seeks to differentiate hemolytic from cholestatic jaundice
      2. Looks at direct and indirect bilirubin
         a. In hemolytic jaundice the predominant bilirubin is unconjugated (indirect)
         b. In cholestatic jaundice the predominant bilirubin is conjugated (direct), as identified by
            i. Finding bilirubin in the urine
            ii. Finding $>\frac{1}{2}$ of serum bilirubin to be direct

II. **Diagnostics**
   A. **History**
      1. Duration of onset
      2. Medications
      3. Drug and alcohol use
      4. Sexual history
      5. Viral prodromal symptoms
      6. Blood disorders or blood transfusions
      7. Family history of cirrhosis or liver disease
      8. Presence of abdominal pain, nausea, vomiting, and/or fever
      9. Presence of itching
      10. Change in color of urine and feces
      11. Systemic symptoms of possible malignant disease
   B. **Examination**
      1. Degree of icterus: scleral, hue of skin color
      2. Signs of chronic liver disease (spider nevi, gynecomastia, testicular atrophy
      3. Abdominal palpation for masses, gallbladder, Murphy's sign

C. **Laboratory data**
  1. **Initial investigations**
     a. CBC and differential and blood smear
     b. Electrolytes, Cr, BUN, glucose
     c. Liver function tests: AST, ALT, alkaline phosphatase, bilirubin
        i. Alkaline phosphatase >2–3 × normal suggests extrahepatic biliary obstruction
        ii. Normal alkaline phosphatase suggests obstruction is unlikely
        iii. High aminotransferase levels, usually >10 × normal, may indicate viral hepatitis or hepatocellular jaundice
     d. Prothrombin time (PT)
     e. Urinalysis for presence of bilirubin (cholestatic)
  2. **For selected patients**
     a. Hepatitis A, B, and/or C serology
     b. Monospot for EBV in young persons
     c. Hemolysis screen
     d. Alcohol level
     e. Antimitochondrial antibody
     f. Other autoimmune serology
  3. **Imaging studies**
     a. **Ultrasound of abdomen**
        i. Evaluates whether or not jaundice is due to extrahepatic cause such as stones in gallbladder or common duct, hepatic lesions, and abnormalities in the head of the pancreas
        ii. Dilatation of common bile duct is missed up to $1/3$ of the time
     b. **CT scan of the abdomen**
        i. Gives information similar to ultrasound
        ii. Much more expensive but may be slightly better in distinguishing between intra- and extrahepatic duct obstruction
  4. **Further evaluation of cholestatic jaundice**
     a. For evaluation of extrahepatic jaundice, refer for percutaneous transhepatic cholangiography or endoscopic retrograde cholangiopancreatography (ERCP)
     b. For evaluation of cholangitis, consider referring directly for ERCP
     c. For evaluation of abnormality in head of pancreas or for defined liver lesion, consider a guided biopsy of lesion
  5. **For suspected hepatocellular disease**
     a. Monitor enzymes and prothrombin time for
        i. Alcohol-induced hepatitis
        ii. Viral hepatitis
     b. Monitoring is usually done on outpatient basis unless patient

     i. Is unable to tolerate food or fluids
    ii. Has fulminant disease and requires aggressive treatment

III. Referral to Gastroenterologist for

A. Uncertainty of diagnosis or treatment
B. Further evaluation of documented or suspected extrahepatic jaundice
C. Monitoring and evaluation of other forms of cholestatic jaundice

Reference

American Gastroenterological Association: Clinical evaluation of jaundice: A guideline of the Patient Care Committee of the American Gastroenterological Association. JAMA 262:3031–3034, 1989.

L

Lower Back Pain

I. General Principles

A. Most episodes (70–90%) of lower back pain resolve within 4–8 wk and will do so no matter what the treatment plan

B. Factors associated with back pain
   1. Heavy labor
   2. Poor posture
   3. Improper lifting technique
   4. Exposure to vibrations
   5. Poor general health
   6. Drug and cigarette abuse
   7. Repetitive work, especially with bending and twisting

C. Occupational back injury is common and costly in dollars and time lost from work

II. Diagnostics

A. **History**
   1. Duration, location, and radiation of pain
   2. Occupational history: lifting, movement, bending
   3. Trauma history
   4. History of cancer
   5. Previous back injuries and treatment
   6. GI and GU systems
   7. Neurologic symptoms
   8. Systemic symptoms: weight loss, malaise, fatigue, fevers
   9. Drug and medication use

B. **Examination**
   1. Palpation of abdomen for masses (e.g., AAA)
   2. Palpation of spine for tenderness (e.g., fracture or localized lesion)
   3. Range of motion of lumbar spine
   4. Power, especially extensor of big toe
   5. Straight leg-raising
   6. Dermatomal sensation testing
   7. Reflexes and Babinski
   8. Breast and thyroid exam, when appropriate
   9. Pelvic exam, when appropriate
   10. Prostate exam in older men

C. **Laboratory data**
   1. **For selected patients**
      a. **X-rays of lumbosacral spine should be considered with**
         i. Neuromotor deficit
         ii. Age >50 y/o

    iii. History of significant trauma

    iv. Pain that has continued unabated for >1 mo

    v. History of alcohol or substance abuse

    vi. Fever and spinal tenderness

    vii. Previous history of malignancy

    viii. Unexplained weight loss or systemic signs of malignancy

    ix. Prolonged corticosteroid use

    x. Suspicion of rheumatologic disease, other than osteoarthritis

    xi. No response to medical treatment after 1 mo

  b. CBC and differential for multiple myeloma

  c. ESR is useful if malignancy or infectious disease is suspected

  d. Urinalysis and/or creatinine, BUN, if renal disease is suspected or prostate exam is abnormal

  e. Calcium and alkaline phosphatase if evaluation suggests bony malignancy or Paget's disease

  f. Acid phosphatase, prostatic-specific antigen if prostate malignancy suspected

  g. Serum and/or urine protein electrophoresis if multiple myeloma suspected

  h. Rheumatoid factor, ANA, HLA, B27, if clinical or x-ray evaluation suggests rheumatologic disease

 2. **Imaging studies**

  a. CT scan of spine can be done with myelogram for suspected cord or radicular impingement syndrome

    i. Spinal stenosis

    ii. Herniated disc

    iii. Malignant disease

  b. MRI is used similarly to CT myelogram

  c. Echocardiography for patient with fever and back pain and clinical suspicion of endocarditis

  d. Bone scan for detection of suspected bony lesions not seen on x-ray

III. **Management**

  A. **General approach to uncomplicated back pain**

   1. **Bedrest**

    a. >2–3 d may not be beneficial

    b. Sleep on firm, back-supporting surface

   2. **Ice**

    a. For first 24–48 hr

    b. Apply for 5–15 min every few hr, while awake

   3. **Heat**

    a. After first 24–48 hr

    b. Heating pads or hot baths

    c. Some recommend alternating with ice

   4. **Massage or whirlpool baths**

5. Avoid lifting and repetitive motion that aggravates LBP
6. **Medications**
    a. **NSAID of choice**
        i. In moderate doses with food
        ii. Limit amount given to avoid side effects of prolonged use
    b. **Muscle relaxant of choice**
        i. If given at all, use short course
            (a) Most patients will not derive much benefit from these after 5–10 d
            (b) These should not be used for maintenance treatment without a formal evaluation from an orthopedist or rheumatologist or other expert on back pain syndromes
            (c) Warn patient about drowsiness
7. **Physical therapy**
    a. Consider referral for assessment and appropriate treatment, including
        i. Program to increase mobility, flexibility, and strength
        ii. Education on proper lifting techniques and posture
        iii. Instruction on home exercises
B. **Chiropractic care by a licensed chiropractic physician**
    1. Chiropractors use massage, traction, mobilization
    2. Physician should be a licensed member of the American Chiropractic Association
    3. Course of treatment is usually 2–4 wk
    4. Spinal manipulation may help those who
        a. Have had relief by manipulation before
        b. Do not want or cannot tolerate drug therapy
        c. Have persistent uncomplicated back pain
        d. Have acute or chronic LBP
    5. Consider referral with
        a. Absence of systemic disease that may affect bony skeleton
        b. No neurologic symptoms
        c. Minor neurologic signs
            i. Asymmetric ankle reflex
            ii. Dermatomal sensory loss
        d. No L/S spine radiographic contraindications
            i. Neoplastic or infectious lesion
            ii. Inflammatory or septic arthritis
            iii. Unhealed fracture
            iv. Local disease (Paget's)
    6. Some patients benefit from chiropractic treatment when they have
        i. Spinal stenosis without neurologic findings
        ii. Herniated disc (nucleus pulposus) with only minor neurologic findings listed above
        iii. Back pain after laminectomy

IV. **Referrals May Include**
  A. Physical therapy, as above
  B. Rheumatology for suspicion of spondyloarthropathy or other rheumatologic disorder
  C. Orthopedic or specialty clinic
    1. For severe chronic or recurrent back pain
    2. If neuromotor deficit found
    3. If spinal stenosis documented or suspected
  D. Chiropractic physician, as above

References

1. Deyo RA, Diehl AK: Cancer as a cause of back pain: Frequency, clinical presentation, and diagnostic strategies. J Gen Intern Med 3:230–238, 1988.
2. Shekelle PG, Adams AH, Chassin MR, et al: Spinal manipulation for low back pain. Ann Intern Med 117:590–598, 1992.

Lung Cancer

I. **General Principles**
  A. **Bronchogenic carcinoma**
    1. Has an incidence of over 150,000 cases/yr
    2. Has overall 5-yr survival rates at 10–15%
    3. Kills over 140,000 persons/yr
    4. Is the commonest fatal malignancy for men and women
    5. Is resectable in only 20–30% of patients
  B. **Solitary pulmonary nodules** (SPN)
    1. Differential diagnosis includes
      a. Solitary primary malignancy
      b. Metastatic disease
      c. Hamartomas
      d. Granulomas
      e. Adenomas
      f. Carcinoid tumors
      g. Organized pneumonia
      h. Pulmonary infarcts
    2. Malignancy is found in about 30–60% of cases
    3. Hamartomas and granulomas may each cause about 5% of SPNs
    4. Up to 20% of small lesions on CXRs may be artifactual
      a. Prior CXRs whenever available are useful
    5. CXR results are generally unreliable for differentiating types of lesions, but malignancy is often associated with
      a. Lesions >3 cm
      b. Calcified spiculations

    c. Lobulated contour
    d. Calcification may be helpful in identifying benign lesions
        i. Granulomas may have
           (a) Dense central nidus
           (b) Diffuse calcification
           (c) Laminated calcification
        ii. Hamartomas may have popcornlike calcification pattern
    e. Prior CXRs may show a long-term stable (e..g, >2 yr) lesion
        i. This almost always indicates benign disease

II. Diagnostics

A. History

1. Smoking history
2. Tuberculosis exposure
3. Family history
4. Respiratory symptoms
   a. Cough with or without production
   b. Hemoptysis
   c. Shortness of breath
   d. Chest pain
5. Systemic symptoms
   a. Fever
   b. Anorexia and/or weight loss
   c. Malaise and fatigue
   d. Neuromuscular complaints
   e. Bony pains
   f. Persistent hoarseness
6. Symptoms for other possible primary sites
   a. Recent change in bowel habit
   b. Breast lumps or discharge
   c. Prostatism or urinary symptoms
   d. Recent testicular enlargement or pain
   e. Pelvic/abdominal pain
   f. Post- or intermenopausal bleeding

B. Examination

1. General: muscular wasting, facial asymmetry
2. Neck examination for masses and/or cervical or supraclavicular lymph node enlargement
3. Respiratory evaluation
4. Breast and axillary node palpation
5. Abdominal palpation for masses and liver enlargement
6. Genital examination
7. Complete neurologic examination
8. Rectal digital examination with guaiac test of stool

C. Laboratory data

1. **Initial investigations**
   a. PA and lateral CXR

      i. Low voltage (70–80 kv) may help to identify calcification

     ii. Some practitioners use conventional tomography and/or fluoroscopy at time of CXR

2. **Further investigations**

  a. CBC and differential

  b. PT and PTT if transthoracic needle biopsy is to be done

  c. Liver function tests, including transaminases, LDH, alkaline phosphates, and bilirubin

  d. Creatinine and BUN

  e. Urinalysis

  f. Pulmonary function tests

  g. **Sputum cytology** has low yield (10–20%) for carcinoma but is helpful if positive

  h. **CT scan should be requested when**

      i. Nature of nodule is indeterminate

     ii. Staging is necessary for suspected malignant disease

    iii. Patient has malignancy that is potentially resectable

      (a) In this case CT evaluation should include thorax and upper abdomen

    iv. Patient has prior history of malignancy

     v. Patient has hilar or mediastinal lymphadenopathy

  i. Thin-section CT with densimetry may be helpful with a

      i. Well-demarcated lesion

     ii Spherical lesion

    iii Lesion <2 cm in diameter

  j. **Bronchoscopy or transthoracic needle biopsy**

      i. Bronchoscopy may be preferred when

      (a) Sputum cytology suggests malignancy

      (b) Nodule >2 cm is contiguous with a bronchus

      (c) Nodule is centrally located

     ii. Transthoracic needle biopsy may be preferred when nodule is

      (a) Peripheral

      (b) <2 cm in diameter

  k. **Thoracotomy and resection** is considered for

      i. Nodules undiagnosed after above diagnostic steps are completed

     ii. Nodules >3 cm without hilar or mediastinal lymph node enlargement by CT scan

    iii. Solitary pulmonary malignancies without evidence of metastatic spread by CT scan or mediastinoscopy or other clinical indications

III. **Management**

A. **General approach**

1. Indeterminate lung lesions in some cases may be watched over time rather than diagnosed by thoracotomy

         a. If so, consider monitoring clinical and CXR features every 2–3 mo for 1 yr, then every 6 mo for second yr, and then yearly thereafter

         b. Refer for thoracotomy if lesion is growing over time

   B. Further management of malignant disease depends on histologic subtype of tumor and stage of disease

      1. Refer management to thoracic surgeon and/or oncologist

   C. Patient and family should be informed of prognosis

IV. **Referral to Oncologist and/or Thoracic Surgeon for**

   A. Uncertainty of diagnosis

   B. Management of suspected or proved malignant disease

   C. Bronchoscopy of other invasive studies

References

1. Khouri NF, Meziane MA, Zerhouni EA, et al: The solitary pulmonary nodule: Assessment, diagnosis, and management. Chest 91:128–133, 1987.
2. Swensen SJ, Jett JR, Payne WS, et al: An integrated approach to evaluation of the solitary pulmonary nodule. Mayo Clin Proc 65:173–186, 1990.

Lyme Disease

I. **Definition**

   A. Lyme disease is a tick-borne disease caused by the spirochete *Borrelia burgdorferi*, which is transmitted by the Ixodes tick

   B. **Case definition** is presence of one of:

      1. **Erythema chronicum migrans**

         a. Annular round red patch with central clearing >5 cm in diameter at site of and/or distant from tick bite, growing in size over a period of days or weeks

      2. **Late manifestations**

         a. Intermittent, self-limited swelling in one or more joints (often involving the knee) and on occasion leading to chronic synovitis (usually 6 or more mo after erythema chronicum migrans)

         b. CNS disorders

            i. Cranial neuritis

            ii. Unilateral or bilateral facial (Bell's) palsy may occur within 1 mo of seroconversion

            iii. Encephalomyelitis

            iv. Meningitis

         c. Myocarditis and/or AV conduction blocks, usually about 1 mo after appearance of rash

II. **General Principles**
   A. Diagnosis is by clinical evaluation of symptoms and signs
      1. Serology is used to provide confirmation of infection
      2. Definitive positive serology is not mandatory for establishing a diagnosis
      3. Late disease without positive serology is rare
   B. To transmit disease tick must usually remain on person for at least 1 d but often a history of tick bite is not found
   C. Most cases occur in Pacific northwest, the northeast, and the upper midwest, but cases can be found throughout most of the U.S.
   D. Endemic areas are those with 2 or more previous cases of Lyme disease or where infected ticks have been found

III. **Diagnostics**

   A. **History**
      1. Exposure to endemic area within last 30 d
      2. History of tick bite
      3. History of annular rash or other recent dermatologic abnormality
      4. Systemic symptoms of fatigue, myalgias
      5. Neurologic symptoms (e.g., Bell's palsy)
      6. Palpitations, lightheadedness
      7. Memory deficits and cognitive changes
   B. **Examination**
      1. Rash
      2. Joint swelling
      3. Facial asymmetry
   C. **Laboratory data**
      1. **Routine**
         a. Lyme titers by ELISA and/or Western blot
         b. **Note:**
            i. False positives may occur with syphilis
            ii. Positive results are **not** necessary for diagnosis of Lyme disease
      2. **For selected patients**
         a. EKG if myocarditis or conduction block suspected
         b. LP if encephalomyelitis or meningitis suspected
            i. This diagnosis must be confirmed by serology on CSF

IV. **Treatment**

   A. **General approach**
      1. When treating carditis, neurologic manifestations other than Bell's palsy, or other severe manifestations of Lyme disease, physicians may wish to consider IV antibiotics and consultation with a specialist
      2. Jarisch-Herxheimer reaction may occur within 24 hr after treatment begins

B. **Treatment regimens** (oral therapy)
   1. For tick bite only
      a. Antibiotics optional but not necessary
      b. Advise patient of Lyme disease manifestations
   2. For asymptomatic seropositivity, no treatment necessary
   3. For early disease (e.g., skin rash) any of
      a. Doxycycline: 100 mg b.i.d. for 10–21 d
      b. Tetracycline: 250 mg q.i.d. for 10–21 d
      c. Erythromycin: 250 mg q.i.d. for 10–21 d
      d. **Note:** Tetracycline is more effective than erythromycin
   4. For facial palsy, treat as per early disease **but** give regimen for 21 d
   5. For neurologic manifestations other than Bell's palsy, use IV therapy with any of
      a. PCN G: 20 MU/d in divided doses
      b. Ceftriaxone: 2 g for 14–21 d
      c. Cefotaxime: 3 g b.i.d. for 14–21 d
   6. For late disease
      a. For arthritis
         i. Doxycycline: 100 mg b.i.d. for 1 mo
         ii. Amoxicillin (500 mg) and probenecid (500 mg) q.i.d. for 1 mo
         iii. Consider IV if severe disease
   7. For carditis, if 1st degree block is present and <0.4 sec, consider
      a. Doxycycline: 100 mg b.i.d. for 21 d
      b. For more severe disease, use IV therapy
C. **Special considerations**
   1. **In pregnant women**
      a. For erythema chronicum migrans (single lesion only)
         i. Amoxicillin: 500 mg t.i.d. for 10–21 d
         ii. PCN VK: 250–500 mg t.i.d. for 10–21 d
      b. For other findings, use IV therapy

V. **Referral to Infectious Disease Specialist for**

   A. Complications of Lyme disease
   B. Uncertainty of diagnostic or treatment guidelines
   C. Negative serologic tests when positive clinical manifestations found

References

1. Malane MS, Grant-Kels JM, Feder HM, Luger SW: Diagnosis of Lyme disease based on dermatologic manifestations. Ann Intern Med 114:490–498, 1991.
2. Rahn DW, Malawista SE: Lyme disease: Recommendations for diagnosis and treatment. Ann Intern Med 114:472–481, 1991.

O

Oral Contraception

I. **General Principles**

   A. More than 50 million women in the U.S. have at one time used the oral contraceptive pill (OCP)

   B. **OCPs are available in the following formulations**
1. Monophasic with constant doses of estrogen and progestin
2. Biphasic and triphasic, with varying doses of estrogen and progestin
3. Progestin only ("minipill"), used rarely today

   C. **Contraindications**
1. Genital bleeding of unknown cause
2. Past or active breast or liver cancers
3. Thromboembolic or vascular disorders
4. Pregnancy

   D. **Precaution should be used with**
1. Asthma
2. Seizures
3. Migraine headaches
4. Renal or hepatic disease
5. Hypertension
6. Hyperlipidemia

   E. **Risk factors** for increased complications
1. Age >40 yr (or >35 yr if patient smokes cigarettes)
2. Familiy history of premature cardiovascular disease
3. Blood pressure $>140/90$ mmHg
4. Diabetes, including gestational
5. Hyperlipidemia
6. Severe migraine headaches
7. Chronic liver disorders
8. Metabolic disorders
9. Tobacco use

   F. **Benefits of OCPs**
1. Reliable contraception when taken properly
2. Regulation of menses
3. Reduction of menorrhagia and dysmenorrhea
4. Decreased risk of benign breast disease, with risk reduction continuing for up to 10 yr after discontinuation of OCP
5. Decreased risk of ovarian and endometrial cancers, with risk reduction continuing for up to 15 yr after discontinuation of OCP

   G. **Adverse effects** include increased risk of

   1. Thromboembolic disease (stroke, MI)
   2. Cholelithiasis
   3. Hepatocellular adenoma
   4. Hypertension

II. Diagnostics

A. History and examination
   1. Evaluation of risk factors listed above
   2. Periodic pelvic examination
B. Laboratory data
   1. **Routine**
      a. Cervical smear every 1–3 years

III. Management

A. General approach
   1. Before prescribing OCP discuss all adverse and beneficial effects with patient
   2. OCP of choice is one with lowest effective dose of hormones
   3. Usual estrogen dose is 30–35 μg/d or as in any of the multiphasic pills
   4. Minor side effects (see below) may diminish over time, but for those that are persistent and bothersome, try different OCP in same estrogen dose range
   5. Over 30 OCPs, with different formulations of sex steroids
      a. Details of hormone type and doses are found below
      b. Consult drug guide for proprietary names
B. Formulations of estrogens and progestins
   1. Estrogens
      a. Mestranol: 50–150 μg
      b. Ethinyl estradiol: 20–50 μg
   2. Progestins
      a. Ethynodiol diacetate: 1 mg
      b. Levonorgestrel: 0.15 mg
      c. Norethindrone: 0.35–2 mg
      d. Norethynodrel: 2.5–9.85 mg
      e. Norethindrone acetate: 1–2.5 mg
      f. Norgestrel: 0.075 mg–0.5 mg
C. Side effects
   1. The following often resolve with continued use
      a. Breakthrough bleeding
      b. Breast swelling and tenderness
      c. Nausea
         i. Advise patient to take pill with food or at bedtime
   2. Alterations in serum levels of
      a. Lipids: HDL and/or LDL may increase or decrease
      b. Thyroid hormones: TBG, T4, and T3 increase
      c. Cortisol, aldosterone, prolactin: increase

D. **Special considerations**
  1. Missed pills
     a. Because of the low dose of estrogen, noncompliance puts patient at risk for pregnancy
     b. Patients who miss pills should be told to use additonal contraception during month at risk
  2. Amenorrhea
     a. OCP-induced amenorrhea is common and need not be corrected unless desired by the patient to feel "normal" or to monitor for pregnancy
     b. If menses are desired, a higher estrogen dose or lower progestin dose may be tried
     c. If pregnancy occurs or is suspected, stop OCP use
  3. Drugs that decrease effectiveness of OCPs
     a. Rifampin
     b. Antiseizure medications: phenobarbital, phenytoin
     c. Antibiotic therapy that alters GI flora
        i. Consider increasing estrogen to 50 μg
  4. Lactation is considered a relative contraindication for use of estrogens and progestin
     a. Some practitioners use the "minipill"
     b. Consult with gynecologist for recommended use
  5. Following discontinuation of OCP, many women may have 1–2 mo of delay before starting regular menses
  6. Women wishing to avoid pregnancy should immediately use other forms of contraception after stopping OCP

IV. **Referral to Gynecologist for**

  A. Uncertainty of management
  B. High-risk patients who desire oral contraceptives
  C. Evaluation of suspected gynecologic disorder
     1. Unexplained genital bleeding
     2. Persistent unexplained amenorrhea
     3. Abnormalities found on pelvic examination

Reference

American College of Obstetrics and Gynecology: Oral Contraception. Am Coll Obstet Gynecol Tech Bull No. 106, July, 1987.

Osteoarthritis

I. **General Principles**
   A. Findings associated with osteoarthritis
      1. Degeneration and reduction of articular cartilage
      2. Subchondral bone and joint margin inflammation
      3. Secondary synovitis
   B. It is important to assess both pain and loss of function from osteoarthritis
   C. Flares of acute inflammation are not uncommon
   D. Joints often affected
      1. Hips and knees
      2. Spine
      3. Distal interphalangeal joints of fingers
      4. Carpometacarpal joint of thumb

II. **Diagnostics**

   A. **History**
      1. Affected joints
      2. Prior joint/limb trauma(s)
      3. Age at onset
      4. Duration and progression of symptoms
      5. Pain is most often dull or throbbing
      6. Joint stiffness should be <30 min
      7. Family history of arthritis
      8. Functional disability
   B. **Examination**
      1. Evaluation of affected joints
         a. Crepitus
         b. Low-grade inflammation
         c. Synovial enlargement
         d. Swelling
         e. Muscle atrophy and/or weakness
         f. Range of motion
      2. Heberden's and/or Bouchard's nodes
   C. **Laboratory data**
      1. **Evaluation of a specific joint**
         a. X-rays of joint
         b. Synovial fluid analysis
         c. Serum uric acid
      2. **For selected patients**
         a. To evaluate possible systemic or other rheumatologic disease
            i. CBC and differential
            ii. ESR or C-reactive protein (CRP)
            iii. Electrolytes and creatinine, BUN

      iv. Rheumatoid factor

      v. Urinalysis

  b. With radicular or neurologic symptoms or signs, consider CT myelogram or MRI

III. Management

A. General approach

1. Analgesics and antiinflammatory agents, when warranted
   a. NSAIDs have significant adverse effects
      i. Use lowest possible effective dose
      ii. Discontinue when not needed to control pain
2. Education regarding range of motion exercises
3. Referral for
   a. Physical therapy
   b. Occupational therapy
   c. Surgical intervention for severe disease
4. Use of cane, walker, or other devices for support and independent living

B. Medical therapy

1. **For acute or low-grade inflammation**
   a. **NSAID of choice**
      i. Short, intermittent courses may reduce adverse profile
      ii. Advise taking with food to minimize gastric upset
      iii. May need to try several different types before patient notes response and/or tolerance
         (a) Trial of medication is usually 14 d before considering switch to other NSAID
         (b) It may be beneficial to choose an NSAID from a different chemical class
   b. Intraarticular corticosteroid injections should be used with caution; physicians may wish to refer to or consult with rheumatologist or orthopedic surgeon
2. **For general aches/pains**
   a. Acetaminophen as needed may be beneficial and tends to have fewer adverse effects
   b. Heating pads or hot soaks for affected areas
   c. Decrease activities that may aggravate condition (e.g., repetitive motion involving affected joints)
   d. Neck collar for support of head
3. **Muscle strengthening and joint stabilizing exercises**
   a. May be helpful for patients with disuse atrophy
   b. Consider referral to physical therapy for assistance in evaluation and advice on exercise program
4. **Functional improvement**
   a. Consider referral to occupational therapy for assistance with functional assessment and evaluating need for assistive devices

C. **Surgical interventions** may include joint replacement, arthro-plasty, and/or arthrodesis
  1. Consider referral to an orthopedic surgeon for
    a. Incapacitation from pain or decreased range of motion of affected joint
    b. Impairment of independent functioning
      i. Toileting and grooming
      ii. Eating and/or cooking
      iii. Bathing
      iv. Dressing
      v. Shopping
      vi. Continence
    a. Inability to engage in fundamental lifestyle
      i. Leisure activities
      ii. Work-related functions
      iii. Sexual activity
      iv. Caring for other person(s)

IV. **Referrrals Should Be Considered for**

  A. Uncertainty of diagnosis of treatment
  B. Undifferentiated rheumatic disease
  C. Evaluation for orthopedic intervention
  D. Evaluation and management by physical and/or occupational therapists

References

1. American College of Rheumatology: Guidelines for Reviewers of Rheumatic Disease Care. Am Coll Rheum 1989, p 12.
2. American Rheumatism Association: Dictionary of Rheumatic Diseases, Vol. II. 1985, pp 88–91.
3. Primer on Rheumatic Diseases, 9th ed. Atlanta, Arthritis Foundation, 1988, pp 171–176.

Osteoporosis

I. **Definition**

Osteoporosis is a disease of progressive bone loss leading to increased bone fragility

II. **General Principles**

A. Osteoporosis affects approximately $1/3$ of postmenopausal women
B. The incidence of osteoporosis-related fractures is estimated at over 1 million/yr

C. **Possible risk factors in women**
   1. White and Asian race
   2. Thin or petite body structure
   3. Family history of osteoporosis
   4. Sedentary lifestyle
   5. Premature menopause
   6. Cigarette smoking, excessive caffeine use, and alcohol abuse
D. **Conditions and diseases that may cause secondary osteoporosis**
   1. Endocrine disorders
      a. Cushing's syndrome
      b. Hyperparathyroidism
      c. Hyperthyroidism
   2. Neoplasia such as multiple myeloma and other hematologic malignancies
   3. Chronic renal failure
   4. Intestinal malabsorption
   5. Medications
      a. Steroids
      b. Anticonvulsants
E. **Use of screening laboratories and imaging studies in asymptomatic women is controversial**
   1. Low- or normal-risk patients usually need only
      a. Education regarding osteoporosis
      b. Advice on diet and exercise
      c. Modification of risk factors
      d. Hormone replacement therapy (HRT), if desired
      e. Periodic monitoring
   2. Women who are already taking or want HRT, no matter what screening or diagnostic studies indicate, do not need screening or diagnostic studies **unless** results will change management
F. **Indications for obtaining screening or diagnostic studies** (see under laboratory data below)
   1. Women who have premature ovarian failure
   2. Women who are incidentally found to have bony changes suggestive of osteoporosis
   3. Women who have symptoms and/or signs of osteoporosis
   4. When consideration for long-term estrogen replacement therapy is predicated on definitive diagnosis of osteoporosis
   5. When studies will change medical management

III. **Diagnostics**

   A. **History**
      1. Presence of risk factors
      2. Dietary history
         a. Intake of vitamin D and calcium
         b. Caffeine intake

        3. Exercise history
        4. Cigarette and alcohol history
        5. Menopausal symptoms, age of onset of menopause

B. **Examination**
        1. Height and weight
        2. Arm span $>$ height suggests significant bone loss has already occurred
        3. Presence of spinal and other bony abnormalities
        4. Presence of signs suggesting secondary causes of osteoporosis

C. **Laboratory data**
        1. **Radiographic screening studies**
            a. Spinal x-rays
                i. Bone loss must be $>20\%$ before abnormalities are seen
            b. Measuring bone densities may include either of
                i. Dual (DPA) or single (SPA) photon absorptiometry
                ii. Quantitative computerized tomography scan
        2. **Evaluation of patient with osteoporosis**
            a. CBC and ESR
            b. Electrolytes, creatinine, and BUN
            c. Calcium, phosphate, and magnesium
            d. Liver function tests, including alkaline phosphatase
            e. 1,25 dihydroxy vitamin D and/or parathyroid hormone
            f. Thyroid studies (if clinically warranted): FT4 (or FTI), TSH
            g. Serum protein electrophoresis
            h. Urinalysis and urinary protein determination
            i. Urine for fasting calcium/creatinine and hydroxyproline/creatinine ratios
            j. 24-hr urine for calcium excretion

IV. **Management**

A. **Prevention**
        1. **Education**
            a. Reduction of modifiable risks (e.g., cigarettes, alcohol)
            b. Diet and exercise advice
        2. **Adequate calcium intake daily**
            a. Young adults: 750–1000 mg q.d.
            b. Premenopausal women over age 30: 1000 mg q.d.
            c. Postmenopausal women: 1,500 mg q.d.
            d. Pregnant women: 1,500 mg q.d.
            e. Lactating women: 2 g q.d.
        3. **Adequate vitamin D intake daily**
            a. Adults: 400 IU q.d.
            b. Elderly: 800 IU q.d.
         4. **Hormone replacement therapy**
            a. For available medications, dosages, and regimens
                • See chapter on "Hormone Replacement Therapy"

       b. Unopposed estrogen therapy can be given safely only if patient has had a hysterectomy

  5. **Monitoring**

    a. Women on estrogen replacement therapy should be monitored periodically

      i. Breast examination (yearly)

      ii. Pelvic examination (every 1–3 yr)

      iii. Blood pressure measurements (yearly)

      iv. Mammography (as indicated)

B. **Treatment for established osteoporosis**

  1. **General approach**

    a. Reduce modifiable risk factors

    b. Diet and exercise advice

      i. Exercise routines should be low impact

    c. Preventative measures against falls at home

      i. Handrails

      ii. Supportive devices

      iii. Avoiding throw rugs or other obstacles

    d. Adequate calcium and vitamin D intake as above

    e. Hormone replacement therapy: estrogens help preserve bone mass

C. **Pharmacotherapy**

  1. Refer to specialist for these options and protocols

V. **Referrals to Endocrinologist or Specialist for**

A. Uncertainty of diagnosis or treatment

B. Rapid, documented bone loss

C. Treatment of established osteoporosis

References

1. American College of Obstetricians and Gynecologists: Osteoporosis. Am Coll Obstet Gynecol Tech Bull No. 118, July, 1988.
2. Consensus Development Conference: Prophylaxis and treatment of osteoporosis. Am J Med 90:107–110, 1991.
3. Editorial: Should prescription of postmenopausal hormone therapy be based on the results of bone densitometry? Ann Intern Med 113:565–567, 1990.
4. Melton LJ, Eddy DM, Johnston CC: Screening for osteoporosis. Ann Intern Med 113:516–528, 1990.

P

Panic Disorder

I. Definition

A. The diagnosis of panic attacks is defined by DSM-III-R as
   1. Discrete periods of intense fear without apparent and known stimulus (e.g., snakes, public speaking, car mishap)
   2. At least 4 of
      a. Shortness of breath or feelings of suffocation
      b. Dizziness, unsteadiness, or faintness
      c. Palpitations or tachycardia
      d. Trembling or shaking
      e. Sweating
      f. Choking
      g. Nausea or abdominal discomfort
      h. Depersonalization or derealization
      i. Paresthesias
      j. Flushes or chills
      k. Chest discomfort or pain
      l. Fear of dying
      m. Fear of going crazy or losing control
   3. Symptoms begin abruptly and reach a crescendo within 10 min
   4. Four such episodes within 4 wk or at least 1 episode followed by 1 mo of dread of another episode

II. General Principles

A. Panic attacks can be debilitating
   1. One-third of sufferers also have agoraphobia
   2. Depression is common
B. Women are affected twice as often as men
C. Onset is often in late adolescence or young adulthood
D. **Conditions that may mimic panic attacks**
   1. Simple and social phobias
      a. Panic in response to feared situation (e.g., snakes, public speaking)
   2. Medication and substance use or withdrawal
      a. Caffeine overdose
      b. Beta agonist use
      c. Cocaine, amphetamines and other stimulants
      d. Alcohol or benzodiazepine use or withdrawal
   3. Other psychiatric disorders
      a. Severe depression
      b. Generalized anxiety syndromes

        4. Organic disease
           a. Asthma
           b. Myocardial ischemia
           c. Pheochromocytoma
           d. Seizure disorder
           e. Hyperthyroidism
           f. Tachyrhythmias
           g. Hypoglycemia

III. **Diagnostics**

A. **History**

1. Age at onset
2. Number of attacks per month
3. Duration of attacks
4. Whether attacks have known precipitants (e.g., fear of a public-speaking engagement)
5. Characteristics of attacks
6. Life events and stressors that may have triggered attacks
7. Previous diagnoses or treatments
8. Family psychiatric history
9. History of physical or mental abuse
10. Drug and alcohol history
11. Symptoms that may be associated with organic disease
    a. Substernal chest pain
    b. Wheezing and cough
    c. Loss of consciousness or altered sensorium
    d. History of hypoglycemic symptoms
    e. Temperature appreciation, general irritability

B. **Examination**

1. Vital signs: hypertension, resting tachycardia
2. General mental state
3. Evaluation of organ systems for signs of above disorders
4. Cardiovascular examination for murmurs and click of MVP
5. Abdomen for masses
6. Neurologic deficits

C. **Laboratory data**

1. **Routine screening**
    a. CBC and differential
    b. Electrolytes, creatinine and BUN
    c. Liver function tests
    d. Calcium and phosphorus
    e. EKG

D. **For selected patients** if one of the following is suspected

1. Pheochromocytoma: urine catecholamine, metanephrines or vanillylmandelic acid
2. MVP with palpitations or other tachyrhythmia: echocardiogram and/or cardiac evaluation
3. Thyroid disorder: TSH
4. Hypoglycemia: evaluation for causes of hypoglycemia

IV. **Management**

A. **General approach**
1. Treatment utilizes either or both of
    a. Psychotherapy: cognitive-behavioral therapy
    b. Medications: tricyclics, benzodiazepines or MAOIs
        i. Benzodiazepines (especially alprazolam) are addictive and, if used, should only be given for short periods of time, possibly while other treatment modalities take effect
2. If single therapy has had no effect within 6–8 wk, consider additional therapeutic modality and/or review diagnosis
3. When successful, therapy is maintained for at least 3–6 mo and then tapered off
4. Urgent treatment and/or referral is needed for
    a. Medical complications of extreme phobias
    b. Fear of undergoing a necessary medical procedure
    c. Generalization of phobic behavior
    d. Impending loss of job or important relationship
    e. Rapid decompensation with potential self-harm

B. **Pharmacologic therapy**
1. **Tricyclic antidepressants**
    a. Are started at low dose and then gradually increased until panic attacks diminish and/or stop
    b. For details on dosage
        • See chapter on "Depression"
    c. Reduction in panic attacks often occurs after about 3–6 wk

2. **Benzodiazepines**
    a. Benzodiazepines have a rapid onset of action but care must be used in discontinuing drug at end of treatment as withdrawal may precipitate panic or panic-like attacks
    b. Benzodiazepines commonly used include
        i. Alprazolam: start at 0.5 mg t.i.d., increase dose at intervals of 3–4 d by 0.5–1 mg/d
            (a) Maintenance dose usually about 2 mg t.i.d.
            (b) Maximum dose is 10 mg/d
        ii. Clonazepam: start at 0.5 mg t.i.d., increase dose as for alprazolam
    c. **Note:** Benzodiazepines are addictive and efficacy of long term use (>4 mo) has not been shown

3. **Other drugs**
    a. MAOI: consult pharmacist, psychiatrist, or drug manual for details of dosage and for warnings on tyramine-containing foods
    b. Beta blockers and clonidine may offer minimal temporary relief but are not particularly useful

V. **Referrals**

   A. Organic disorders or other psychiatric disorders are referred appropriately

   B. A psychiatrist or specialist in panic disorders is appropriate for
      1. Uncertainty of diagnosis or treatment
      2. For psychotherapy
      3. Failure of good response from drug therapy

References

1. National Institutes of Health: Treatment of Panic Disorder. Washington, DC, DHHS, 1991.
2. Raj A, Sheehan DV: Medical evaluation of panic attacks. J Clin Psychiatry 48:309–313, 1987.

Pelvic Inflammatory Disease

I. **Definition**

   A. Pelvic inflammatory disease (PID) is a term encompassing
      1. Salpingitis and salpingo-oophoritis
      2. Endomyometritis
      3. Pelvic peritonitis
      4. Tuboovarian abscesses

II. **General Principles**

   A. Incidence of PID is approximately 1 million cases/yr

   B. Most PID is caused by ascending spread of organisms from vagina

   C. Women with a history of PID have **greater risk for**
      1. Ectopic pregnancy
      2. Tubal infertility
      3. Chronic pelvic pain

   D. Most cases of PID are caused by **more than 1 species,** including
      1. *Neisseria gonorrhoeae*
      2. *Chlamydia trachomatis*
      3. Anaerobic bacteria (*Bacteroides, Peptococcus*)
      4. Aerobic bacteria (*Gardnerella,* gram-negative rods)

   E. Those at **higher risk of PID** include
      1. Sexually active adolescents
      2. Persons with multiple partners
      3. Persons with new partner within past month

   F. **Routine screening for asymptomatic chlamydial and gonococcal infection** should be considered for
      1. Sexually active adolescents, especially females
      2. Prostitutes

3. Drug and substance abusers
4. Pregnant women

III. **Diagnostics**

A. **History**
1. Symptoms of PID
   a. Vaginal discharge
   b. Abdominal pain and/or mass
   c. Fevers and chills
   d. Dysuria
   e. Dyspareunia (superficial or deep)
2. Symptoms of STD in partner(s)
3. Rectal or oral symptoms
4. Gynecologic history
   a. Type of contraception used
   b. Menstrual cycle and last menses
   c. Number of recent partners

B. **Examination**
1. Temperature: often >38.3 C
2. Abdominal tenderness and/or masses
3. Bilateral adnexal tenderness
4. Cervical motion tenderness
5. Vaginal or mucopurulent cervical discharge

C. **Laboratory data**
1. **Routine**
   a. Cultures of cervical secretions: *N. gonorrhoeae, C. trachomatis*
   b. Evaluation of discharge: wet mount, potassium hydroxide (KOH) preparation and/or gram stain
   c. Pregnancy test (urine)
2. **For selected patients** or if diagnosis uncertain
   a. Syphilis serology if gonorrhea or chlamydia suspected
   b. Urinalysis if dysuria or UTI suspected
   c. CBC with differential
   d. ESR or C-reactive protein
   e. Ultrasound if abscess suspected on examination
   f. Laparoscopy if diagnosis uncertain

IV. **Management**

A. **General approach**
1. Have a low threshold for admission for IV antibiotics
2. **Follow-up outpatients within 48–72 hr**
   a. If no improvement, reconsider diagnosis and/or consider hospitalization
3. HIV-infected and immunosuppressed women are at higher risk for serious sequelae
   a. Monitor closely if outpatient therapy given

    4. Hospitalize for further diagnostics and/or IV antibiotics if
       a. The diagnosis is uncertain
       b. Surgical emergency, peritonitis, or abscess is suspected
       c. Patient cannot tolerate or follow an outpatient regimen for any reason
       d. Patient is pregnant or an adolescent
       e. There has been no response to outpatient therapy

B. Outpatient treatment (for other regimens consult antibiotic guide or specialist)
    1. **One** of the following
       a. Cefoxitin (2 g IM) **and** probenecid (1 g PO)
          or
       b. Ceftriaxone: 250 mg IM
    2. And **one** of
       a. Doxycycline: 100 mg PO b.i.d. for 10–14 d
       b. Tetracycline: 500 mg PO q.i.d. for 10–14 d
       c. Erythromycin: 500 mg PO q.i.d. for 10–14 d
          i. Erythromycin used only if patient is allergic to or cannot tolerate doxycycline/tetracycline

C. **Special considerations**
    1. Instructions and education
       a. Abstain from sex while patient or partner(s) is being treated
       b. Danger of HIV infection from unprotected sexual intercourse
    2. Diagnosis of PID is indication for removal of IUD
    3. **Sexual partners**
       a. If patient is found to have gonorrhea or chlamydia, then treat partners empirically for gonorrhea or chlamydia

V. **Referral to Gynecologist and/or STD Clinic for**

A. Uncertainty of diagnosis or management
B. Specialized diagnostics
C. Follow-up treatment and/or monitoring
D. Treatment for partner(s)
E. Complications from PID

Reference

Centers for Disease Control: Pelvic inflammatory disease: Guidelines for prevention and management. MMWR 40:1–25, 1991.

Peptic Ulcer Disease

I. **Definition**
 A. Dyspepsia refers to epigastric symptoms such as
  1. Pain
  2. Discomfort and bloating
  3. Nausea and/or vomiting
  4. Early satiety
  5. Gaseousness
  6. Difficulty in tolerating fatty foods or a full meal

II. **General Principles**
 A. Dyspepsia may be divided into the following classifications
  1. Gastric ulcer
  2. Duodenal ulcer
  3. Gastric cancer
  4. Other: noncancer, nonulcer causes
   • Refer also to chapter on "Heartburn and Indigestion"
 B. Up to 20% of people with dyspepsia may have an ulcer
 C. Less than 1% will turn out to have cancer
 D. Most have gastritis, duodenitis, reflux esophagitis (see chapter on "Esophageal Disorders" for details) or no obvious cause
 E. Most gastric ulcers ($2/3$) heal spontaneously by 12 wk

III. **Diagnostics**
 A. **History**
  1. Duration, timing, type, and radiation of pain/discomfort
  2. Association with food or types of food
  3. Relief with food or certain medications (e.g., antacids)
  4. Weight loss: amount lost over time
  5. Nausea and vomiting
  6. Bowel habits: melanic stool, bloody stool
  7. Systemic symptoms: weakness, fatigue
  8. Medications: NSAIDs, aspirin or aspirin-containing preparations, steroids
  9. Alcohol and smoking histories
  10. Amount of coffee and caffeinated beverages (promotes gastric reflux)
  11. Previous diagnoses or treatment of ulcer disease
 B. **Examination**
  1. Eyes: icterus, pale conjunctiva
  2. Mouth: ulcerations, dentition
  3. Neck: lymphadenopathy (supraclavicular)
  4. Abdomen: for masses, tenderness
  5. Rectal: for stool hemoccult

C. **Laboratory data**
  1. **For selected patients**
      a. CBC and indices
          i. If guaiac is positive
          ii. If anemia is suggested by clinical evaluation
      b. Liver function tests if underlying liver disease suspected
  2. Imaging modalities
      a. Ultrasound if gallbladder stones suspected
      b. Endoscopy (EGD) with biopsy
      c. Upper gastrointestinal (double contrast) barium series

IV. **Management**

  A. **General approach**
  1. Evaluate and reduce behaviors that may worsen dyspepsia
      a. Alcohol
      b. Cigarettes
      c. Nonsteroidal medications
      d. Other ulcerogenic drugs
      e. Caffeinated beverages
  2. Combination of ulcer-healing drugs (see below) has not been shown to be more effective than use of single drug
  3. **Complicated dyspepsia** (see below) should be evaluated by an imaging procedure
      a. Endoscopy is preferred but if unavailable or delayed, consider upper GI series
      b. Complicated dyspepsia is epigastric symptoms and one or more of
          i. Weight loss
          ii. Severe systemic illness or evidence of cancer
          iii. GI bleeding
          iv. Gastric obstruction
          v. Dysphagia or persistent vomiting
              • **Note:** many practitioners first request a barium study for evaluation of dysphagia
  4. Uncomplicated dyspepsia is often given a trial of medication of 6–8 wk before deciding on need for further evaluation

  B. **With uncomplicated dyspepsia consider**
  1. **Empirical therapy for 6–8 weeks**
      a. Antacids
          i. Aluminum and magnesium hydroxide compounds such as
              (a) Maalox TC or Mylanta II
                  (i) 15 ml (1 tbs) q.i.d., 30 min after meals q.h.s.
              (b) Gelusil
          ii. Magnesium hydroxide compounds, such as
              (a) Milk of magnesia
          iii. Aluminum hydroxide compounds, such as
              (a) Amphojel or Riopan

          iv. Calcium carbonate compounds, such as
             (a) Tums
     b. H_2 blockers (in alphabetical order)
          i. Cimetidine (Tagamet): 400 mg b.i.d. or 800 mg q.h.s.
          ii. Famotidine (Pepcid): 20 mg b.i.d. or 40 mg q.h.s.
          iii. Nizatidine (Axid): 150 mg b.i.d. or 300 mg q.h.s.
          iv. Ranitidine (Zantac): 150 mg b.i.d. or 300 mg q.h.s.
     c. Other
          i. Carafate (sucralfate): 1 g q.i.d.
             (a) Take on an empty stomach
             (b) Avoid concurrent antacids
          ii. Metoclopramide (Reglan): 10 mg t.i.d.
             (a) Increases gastric emptying
             (b) Take 30 min before meals
             (c) Not often used alone for dyspepsia
          iii. Omeprazole (Prilosec): 20 mg q.d.
             (a) This is an expensive drug indicated for
                (i) Severe erosive esophagitis
                (ii) Severe or refractory duodenal ulcers
                (iii) Zollinger-Ellison syndrome
          iv. Misoprostol (Cytotec): 200 μg q.i.d.
             (a) For protection of gastric mucosa for those at high risk of gastric ulcer (i.e., elderly on NSAID treatment)
     d. Considerations
          i. Some antacids are very high in sodium and care should be taken when prescribing these to
             (a) Persons who are on a low sodium diet
             (b) Persons who have CHF, renal failure, cirrhotic liver disease

  2. **Endoscopy should be strongly considered** if patient has
     a. No response to therapy after 7–10 d
     b. Complication of ulcer disease
     c. Persisting symptoms despite 6–8 wk of compliance with medical treatment
     d. Recurrence of symptoms after medical treatment
  3. **If upper GI series is imaging procedure first used**
     a. Treatment may be based on finding of benign ulcer disease
     b. Refer for EGD and biopsies if
          i. Findings are suspicious for malignancy or other serious underlying problem
          ii. Medical treatment as based on upper GI series is unsuccessful

V. **Referral to Gastroenterologist for**

  A. Indications listed above
  B. Urgent endoscopic examination
  C. Uncertainty of diagnosis or management

References

1. American College of Physicians: Endoscopy in the evaluation of dyspepsia. Ann Intern Med 102:266–269, 1985.
2. Hixson LJ, Kelly CL, Jones WN, Touhy CD: Current trends in the pharmacotherapy for peptic ulcer disease. Arch Intern Med 152:726–733, 1992.

Peripheral Vascular Disease

I. **General Principles**

   A. Prevalence by age group of peripheral vascular disease (PVD) with intermittent claudication
      1. <60 y/o is about 2%
      2. From 60–70 y/o is about 4%
      3. >70 y/o is above 5%
   B. Men are affected twice as often as women
   C. **Risk factors**
      1. Similar to cardiovascular disease
      2. Diabetics are particularly affected
      3. Cigarette smoking may be most important risk
   D. The majority (75%) of those affected
      1. Have stable symptoms over the long term
      2. Die because of coronary disease
   E. **Categories of disease** are generally classified as
      1. Femoropopliteal
      2. Tibioperoneal
      3. Aortoiliac

II. **Diagnostics**

   A. **History**
      1. Duration and progression of symptoms
         a. Rest or nocturnal pain
         b. Reproducibility of pain on exercise
      2. Distance patient can walk until pain begins
      3. Assessment of risk factors
         a. Cigarette smoking
         b. Hypercholesterolemia
         c. Diabetes
         d. Hypertension
      4. Medications
      5. Symptoms of myocardial ischemia
      6. Impotence or sexual dysfunction
   B. **Examination**
      1. Abdominal exam for aortic aneurysm
      2. Vascular exam for palpable pulses and bruits, especially over abdomen and femoral arteries

3. Skin changes in limb(s)
   a. Atrophic skin and/or brittle nails
   b. Ulcerations and gangrene
   c. Hair loss
4. Presence of "blue-toe" syndrome
5. Assessment of other possible causes of leg pain
   a. Spinal stenosis
   b. Arthritis
   c. Sciatic pain

C. **Laboratory data**
   1. **Noninvasive tests**
      a. **Ankle/brachial index (ABI)**
         i. Usually the baseline test for suspected PVD
         ii. Ankle systolic pressure is divided by arm pressure
            (a) Normal ratio is 0.9 or above
            (b) Claudication usually occurs at 0.5–0.9
            (c) Rest pain usually occurs when ratio <0.5
      b. **Segmental blood pressure measurements**
         i. Are at least 2 sequential BP measurements taken at different locations on the same extremity and are used once ABI ratio indicates possibility of PVD
         ii. A drop of 20 mmHg between measurement positions indicates likely location of occlusive lesion
         iii. Can also be used to compare BP of both limbs
            (a) A 20-mmHg difference between similar sites indicates likely location of occlusion
      c. **Treadmill walking test**
         i. Useful for documenting functional disability of PVD and for assessing possible PVD in patients who have normal ABI
         ii. Exercise should cause ankle pressure to drop
            (a) If no reduction occurs, consider spinal stenosis or other cause of leg pain
         iii. Duration and magnitude of decrease indicate severity of disease
      d. **Doppler or duplex scanning** can be used to
         i. Detect type and length of occlusion
         ii. Help localize the site of the lesion (e.g., aortoiliac or femoral)
      e. **Plethysmography** to assess toe/brachial pressure index
         i. Useful for documenting severity of distal disease
         ii. Toe/brachial index ratio
            (a) <0.6 is abnormal
            (b) <0.15 suggests poor healing of distal ulcers
      f. **Angiography**
         i. Use when assessing patients for possible surgical intervention

III. **Management**
   A. **General approach**
      1. **If ABI ratio is 0.9 or higher**
         a. Arterial disease is unlikely; consider alternative disorder
         b. If symptoms strongly suggest PVD, consider treadmill test or Doppler exam to help document occlusive disease
      2. **If ABI ratio indicates likelihood of disease**
         a. Use segmental BP measurements or ultrasound to locate occluded segments of artery
         b. Refer for evaluation by vascular surgeon if
            i. Impending or actual limb-threatening ischemia
            ii. Disabling claudication
            iii. Rest pain
            iv. Complication of arterial disease, including ulceration or gangrenous changes
            v. Noninvasive tests detect aortoiliac disease
         c. If surgical intervention not required, treat conservatively
   B. **Conservative management** for mild to moderate intermittent claudication
      1. Cessation of smoking (a must)
      2. Gradually increasing exercise program (walking or cycling)
      3. Monitor and treat hypertension
      4. Control hyperlipidemia and diabetes
      5. Weight reduction if overweight
      6. Careful foot and skin care
      7. Optimize other comorbid medical problems such as CHF, COPD
      8. Medications
         a. Aspirin: 325 mg q.i.d.
            i. Controversial as to whether it effects PVD
            ii. Often recommended because of cardio- and cerebrovascular disease associated with PVD
         b. Pentoxifylline (Trental): 400 mg t.i.d.
            i. Controversial as to whether it is effective
            ii. Decrease dose to 400 mg b.i.d. if GI upset occurs
      9. Consider appropriate evaluation if
         a. Symptoms indicate cardio- or cerebrovascular disease such as TIAs
         b. Patient has carotid bruit (see chapter on "Carotid Stenosis and Bruits")
      10. If patient is to undergo surgery, evaluate appropriately
         • See chapter on "Preoperative Assessment: Cardiac Risks of Noncardiac Surgery"

IV. **Referrals to Vascular Surgeon for**
   A. Uncertainty of diagnostics or management
   B. Invasive interventions (indications as above)

C. Aortoiliac disease
D. Complications of vascular disease

References

1. Barnes RW: Noninvasive diagnostic assessment of peripheral vascular disease. Circulation 83(Suppl 1):I-20–I-27, 1991.
2. Editorial: Intermittent claudication—Be conservative. N Engl J Med 325:577–578, 1991.
3. Nicolaides AN: Assessment of leg ischaemia. Br Med J 303:1326–1328, 1991.
4. Wilt TJ: Current strategies in the diagnosis and management of lower extremity peripheral vascular disease. J Gen Intern Med 7:87–101, 1992.

Polymyalgia Rheumatica and Giant Cell Arteritis

I. Definition

A. Polymyalgia rheumatica (PMR) refers to a clinical syndrome of severe achiness and stiffness of the shoulder and/or pelvic girdle
B. Etiology is unknown

II. General Principles

A. Prevalence is primarily in persons >50 y/o
B. Twice as many women as men are affected
C. **Principal manifestations**
   1. Achiness and stiffness, especially in the morning or after inactivity
   2. Arthralgias
   3. Synovitis and joint swelling
   4. Systemic symptoms: fever, malaise, low-grade fever
D. Giant cell (temporal) arteritis (GCA) can occur alone or with polymyalgia (10–15%)
E. PMR and GCA are self-limited disorders, with resolution usually within 6–24 mo

III. Diagnostics

A. History

   1. Eliciting symptoms above
      a. Difficulty doing activities because of achiness/stiffness
      b. Difficulty in rolling over in bed
      c. Inability to stand on toes and stretch upward
   2. Evaluating presence of giant cell arteritis
      a. Headache
      b. Severe tenderness over temporal region

        c. Jaw claudication
        d. Sudden loss of vision
        e. Systemic symptoms are similar to those of PMR
  B. **Examination**
      1. Musculoskeletal
        a. True muscle weakness is absent
        b. Periarticular tenderness
        c. Low-grade synovitis
      2. Arterial palpation
        a. Tender, firm temporal arteries
      3. Arterial auscultation
        a. Bruits over arteries sometimes may be heard in GCA
  C. **Laboratory data**
      1. Initial investigations may include
        a. ESR or C-reactive protein are almost always very high
        b. CBC sometimes shows mild anemia
        c. Serum total protein and albumin may be low
        d. Urinalysis for red cells and red cell casts (for vasculitis)
        e. Electrolytes and Cr, BUN
        f. Rheumatoid factor
      2. For selected patients some practitioners suggest
        a. Aminotransferases: SGOT/SGPT
        b. CPK
      3. If giant cell arteritis suspected, request
        a. Temporal biopsy
        b. EKG

IV. **Management**

  A. **For mild PMR** without significant laboratory abnormalities
      1. NSAID of choice
      2. Analgesics
      3. Patient education regarding symptoms of GCA
  B. **For more severe PMR or PMR not responsive to NSAIDs**
      1. **Moderate dose of oral corticosteroids**
        a. Begin at prednisone 10–30 mg q.d. (or equivalent corticosteroid)
        b. Once PMR controlled (usually about 4 wk), reduce dose by about 10%/wk to the minimum necessary to keep symptoms under control
        c. Education about symptoms of GCA
  C. **For suspected temporal arteritis**
      1. **Immediately** begin prednisone (60–80 mg q.d.) or equivalent and refer urgently for temporal artery biopsy
      2. Note: if patient has visual symptoms, start at 80 mg q.d.
  D. **Monitoring PMR and GCA**
      1. See again every 1–4 wk, depending on severity of disease, until stable
      2. Once stable, every 3–6 mo until remission

3. Monitor laboratory data as needed for symptoms/signs
   a. ESR is usually used to monitor disease and adjust dose of steroids
4. If patient is on high-dose steroids, periodically monitor CBC, serum K, glucose, and tonometry
5. Once in presumed remission, taper steroids and watch for relapse of symptoms

V. **Referral to Rheumatologist for**

A. Uncertainty of diagnosis or treatment
B. Monitoring of treatment for PMR and/or GCA
C. Other rheumatologic disorders

References

1. American College of Rheumatology: Guidelines for reviewers of rheumatic disease care. American College of Rheumatology, 1989.
2. American Rheumatism Association: Dictionary of the Rheumatic Diseases. Vol. II: Diagnostic Testing. 1985, pp 88–91.
3. Arthritis Foundation: Primer on Rheumatic Diseases, 9th ed. Atlanta, Arthritis Foundation, 1988, pp 134–135.

Prostatism: Benign Hyperplasia and Cancer Screening

I. **General Principles**

A. Prostatism usually occurs in men >50 y/o
B. Usual causes
   1. Benign prostatic hyperplasia (BPH)
   2. Acute and chronic prostatitis
   3. Prostatic carcinoma
C. The incidence of prostate cancer is approximately 130,000 per year
D. Yearly rectal examination is indicated in men >50 y/o to evaluate size and symmetry of prostate gland
E. There is no consensus on how and when to use prostate-specific antigen (PSA) in screening for prostatic carcinoma
   1. Recent opinion indicates that PSA should be used in conjunction with digital rectal examination (DRE)
   2. **Note:** DRE alone may miss about $1/3$ of early prostatic carcinomas, whereas PSA alone may miss $1/5$ of palpable tumors
F. Characteristic presentation of prostatism
   1. Hesitancy in starting urination
   2. Reduced flow of urine
   3. Dribbling at end of urination

G. BPH may result in
   1. Recurrent urinary tract infections
   2. Obstructive renal failure
H. Symptoms of BPH often remain stable or occasionally improve without treatment

II. **Diagnostics**
   A. **History**
      1. Assessment of presence of
         a. Hesitancy, poor flow, and dribbling
         b. Nocturia
         c. Urgency
         d. Daytime frequency
         e. Feeling of incomplete emptying of bladder
         f. Infection
         g. Pelviperineal pain
         h. Lower back ache and other bony pains of recent onset
      2. **Medications that may worsen or precipitate prostatism**
         a. Anticholinergics: antihistamines, tricyclics
         b. Antispasmodics: propantheline, atropine
         c. Sympathomimetics (often included in "cold" medicines): Pseudoephedrine, phenylpropanolamine, terbutaline, metaproterenol
         d. Diuretics
   B. **Examination**
      1. Abdominal and flank exam for
         a. Palpable bladder
         b. Renal mass
      2. DRE
         a. For size, symmetry, and nodularity of prostate
         b. Tenderness
   C. **Laboratory data**
      1. **Initial investigations**
         a. Urinalysis (and culture, if white cells, hematuria or bacteriuria seen)
         b. Cr and BUN
      2. **Further investigations**
         a. CBC and differential with hematuria or renal mass or for suspected infection
         b. Postvoid residual if bladder obstruction likely
            i. Normal: <50 ml
            ii. Abnormal: ≥200 ml
            iii. Inconclusive: 50–199 ml
         c. Acid phosphatase (AP) if prostate examination suspicious for tumor
         d. PSA
            i. If prostate examination is suspicious for a tumor
            ii. When used in combination with DRE for screening
            iii. May be elevated with BPH or prostatitis

iv. $>4.0\ \mu g/L$ is elevated, but $>10.0\ \mu g/ml$ is markedly elevated and suggests carcinoma

e. Imaging studies
   i. Rectal ultrasound: for sizing prostatic enlargement and assessing potential for invasive carcinoma
      (a) Highest sensitivity and specificity when used in conjunction with DRE and PSA
   ii. Ultrasound of kidneys: if hydronephrosis suspected
      (a) Palpable mass
      (b) Decreased renal function
   iii. Intravenous urogram (IVU) may be indicated if
      (a) Renal stone disease suspected
      (b) Hematuria is present
      (c) Recurrent UTI
      (d) Hydronephrosis without bladder obstruction

III. Management

A. General approach

1. Patients with DRE suspicious for carcinoma (e.g., nodule palpated) are referred to a urologist, no matter what the PSA or AP result(s)
2. When DRE and PSA are used for screening, the following methodology should be considered
   a. If both examination and PSA are normal
      i. Follow patient yearly with DRE and PSA
   b. If DRE is normal, but PSA is 4.1–10.0 $\mu g/L$
      i. Request transrectal ultrasound
      ii. Refer to urologist for further assessment
   c. If DRE is normal, but PSA is $>10..0\ \mu g/L$
      i. Request transrectal ultrasound
      ii. Refer to urologist for
         (a) Probable biopsy of suspicious lesion if found
         (b) Systematic biopsy if no lesion is seen
3. If patient suspected of having prostatitis
   a. Treatment may greatly reduce prostatic symptoms
   b. See chapter on "Prostatitis" for further details
4. Once benign disease is diagnosed
   a. Discuss options for treatment
   b. Describe potential risks and complications of surgery and nonsurgical treatment
   c. Reduce or avoid drugs or substances that may worsen prostatic symptoms

B. Nonsurgical management of BPH

1. **Observations**
   a. Many patients and physicians elect to monitor progression, if any, of symptoms
2. **Drugs to be avoided,** if possible
   a. Anticholinergics: antihistamines, tricyclics

b. Antispasmodics: propantheline, atropine
c. Sympathomimetics: pseudoephedrine, phenylpropanolamine, terbutaline, metaproterenol
d. Diuretics: if needed, give in morning to reduce nocturia
3. Avoid or reduce beverage consumption late in evening
4. Minimize coffee, tea, and alcohol
5. **Pharmaceutical therapy**
   a. Drug therapy to reduce prostate size includes
      i. Prazosin: 1–2 mg b.i.d.
      ii. Terazosin: 2–5 mg q.d.
      iii. Finasteride 5 mg q.d.
   b. Once on medical therapy, monitor patient at least yearly for
      i. Worsening of symptoms
      ii. Complications of BPH (e.g., recurrent UTI)
C. **Surgical**
   1. Usual methods are transurethral (TURP) or open surgery
      a. Open surgery is usually for very large glands
   2. **About TURP**
      a. Reduction or stabilization of symptoms occurs 70–90% of time
      b. Reoperation rate (for recurrent symptoms) is about 2% per year
      c. Complications may include
         i. Fluid overload from bladder irrigation causing hyponatremia
         ii. Postoperative infection or bleeding
         iii. Urethral stricture: risk <10%
         iv. Incontinence: less than 5% of patients have permanent incontinence
         v. Impotence: at higher risk are men with reduced potency preoperatively
         vi. Mortality
            (a) For most average-risk patients: <0.2%
            (b) For fragile patients, especially >80 y/o: 5% or higher

IV. **Referral to Urologist for**
   A. Potential or suspected malignant disease
   B. Uncertainty of diagnosis or management
   C. Surgical and advanced diagnostic procedures
   D. Help in starting medical management as an alternative to surgical intervention

References

1. American Urological Association: Guidelines for Urologic Patient Care. AUA, 1987, pp 10–17.
2. Editorial: Prostate-specific antigen: Improving its ability to diagnose early prostate cancer. JAMA 267:2236–2238, 1992.

3. Gittes RF: Carcinoma of the prostate. N Engl J Med 324:236–244, 1991.
4. Stimson JB, Fihn SD: Benign prostatic hypertrophy and its treatment. J Gen Intern Med 5:153–164, 1990.

Prostatitis

I. **Definition**

    A. Prostatitis is inflammation of the prostate and has both bacterial and nonbacterial causes

II. **General Principles**

    A. Clinically significant prostatitis usually occurs when 10 or more white cells per high powered field are seen in prostatic fluid

    B. Prostatitis may be classified as
        1. Acute
        2. Chronic
        3. Nonbacterial: acute or chronic

    C. Nonbacterial prostatitis is a sterile culture and prostatic secretions with 1000 or more white cells per ml or a tenfold increase of urinary white cells after prostatic massage

    D. Prostatic pain and symptoms without evidence of inflammation is known as prostatodynia

    E. **Causative agents**
        1. Bacterial prostatitis is most often caused by
            a. *E. coli* and other gram-negative bacteria
            b. *Enterococcus*
        2. Nonbacterial prostatitis may be caused by
            a. *Chlamydia trachomatis*
            b. *Ureaplasma urealyticum*
            c. Idiopathic causes

    F. Symptoms of acute bacterial prostatitis
        1. Fever and lower back, perineal, or testicular pain
        2. Urinary frequency, dysuria
        3. Obstructive symptoms: hesitancy, poor stream, dribbling
        4. Malaise and fatigue

    G. Symptoms of chronic bacterial prostatitis
        1. Intermittent and recurrent bacteriuria
        2. Sometimes with pelvic or perineal pain
        3. Chronic obstructive symptoms

    H. Symptoms of nonbacterial prostatitis
        1. Pelvic, low back, perineal, and/or testicular pain
        2. Chronic obstructive symptoms

III. **Diagnostics**

    A. **History**
        1. Onset and duration of symptoms
        2. Previous episodes of prostatitis

3. Previous antibiotic or other treatment
4. Prostatic and systemic symptoms
5. Frequency, dysuria, hematuria
6. Penile discharge
7. Recent procedures, (i.e., catheterization)

B. **Examination**
   1. Abdominal and flank exam
   2. Urethral examination for discharge
   3. Rectal exam looking for
      a. Hard, tender, hot, irregular-shaped prostate gland
      b. Fluctuance

C. Laboratory data
   1. **Routine**
      a. Urinalysis and culture
      b. Urine leukocytes per high power field
   2. **For selected patients**
      a. For patients with penile discharge: urethral swabs and cultures
      b. For patients with recurrent prostatitis and nondiagnostic urinalysis
         i. Gram stain and culture of prostatic secretions
         ii. Analysis of urine samples before and after "milking" prostate
            • See "V. Helpful Techniques," below

IV. **Management**

A. **General approach**
   1. Attempt to identify organism, especially in chronic bacterial prostatitis
      • See "V. Helpful Techniques," below
   2. In young men, men with new sexual partners, and men whose cultures are negative for bacteria, consider *Ureaplasma* or *Chlamydia* as etiological agents
   3. Toxic patients need IV antibiotics
   4. Prostatic abscesses need incision and drainage

B. **For acute prostatitis**
   1. In patients suspected of having *Ureaplasma* or *Chlamydia* or in a man <40 y/o, consider using one of
      a. Doxycycline: 100 mg b.i.d. for 2–4 wk
      b. Tetracycline: 500 mg q.i.d. for 2–4 wk
   2. In a male 40 y/o or older, consider using one of
      a. Trimethoprim/sulfamethoxazole: 160/800 mg b.i.d. for 2–4 wk
      b. Amoxicillin: 500 mg t.i.d. for 2–4 wk
      c. Or oral cephalosporin of choice for 2–4 wk

C. **For chronic bacterial prostatitis,** consider using any of
   1. Trimethoprim/sulfamethoxazole as above for 12 wk
   2. Ciprofloxacin: 500 mg b.i.d. for 12 wk
   3. Norfloxacin: 400 mg b.i.d. for 12 wk

D. **For nonbacterial prostatitis**
  1. Consider treatment for *Chlamydia* or *Ureaplasma*
  2. Symptomatic treatment includes NSAID of choice for 1–2 wk and hot sitz baths
E. **Follow-up**
  1. Patients should be followed by urinalysis and culture to ensure clearance of organism and white cells
  2. Recurrent prostatitis needs evaluation of prostatic secretions
     • See "V. Helpful Techniques," below
  3. In some cases of recurrent bacterial prostatitis suppressive therapy may be given
     a. Consult or refer to urologist for details
  4. Underlying carcinoma of the prostate should be considered if repeated prostate exams indicate persistence of a hard and irregular gland after treatment

V. **Helpful Techniques**

  A. **To obtain prostatic secretions**
    1. Digitally massage prostate
    2. Milk urethra
    3. Send specimen for Gram stain, quantitative leukocyte count, and culture
  B. **To obtain serial urine sample**
    1. Sample first 10–20 ml of urine and stop urine flow
    2. Digitally massage prostate
    3. Sample next 10–20 ml of urine
    4. Allow urine flow to clear urethra
    5. Sample last 10–20 ml of urine
    6. Send samples for gram analysis, Gram stain, quantitative leukocyte count, and culture

VI. **Referral to Urologist for**

  A. Uncertainty of diagnosis or treatment
  B. Failure of medical therapy
  C. Persistent irregularity of prostate gland
  D. Persistent or worsening symptoms of prostatism
  E. Persistent pelvic/perineal pain
  F. Symptoms of prostatitis without evidence of inflammation or infection

References

1. Harrison's Principles of Internal Medicine, 12th ed. New York, McGraw-Hill, 1991, pp 543–544.
2. Schaeffer AJ: Diagnosis and treatment of prostatic infections. Urology November(Suppl):13–17, 1990.

R

Renal Stones

I. **General Principles**

    A. Incidence of renal stones (nephrolithiasis) is approximately 70–210 cases/100,000 persons

    B. Men are affected 4× more frequently than women

    C. Onset usually occurs between ages 20–30 y/o

    D. Approximately 60% of those with renal stones will not have another stone for at least 10 yr

    E. **Stones may consist of**

        1. **Calcium oxalate** (70–80% of stones), which may be associated with

            a. Hyperparathyroidism

            b. Renal tubular acidosis

            c. Sarcoidosis

            d. Vitamin D intoxication

            e. Idiopathic hypercalciuria

            f. Low urinary citrate (e.g., in bowel disease)

            g. Medications

        2. Calcium phosphate

        3. Struvite (magnesium ammonium, phosphate) stones may occur with infection by urea-splitting bacteria (e.g., *Proteus*)

        4. Uric acid

            a. From hyperuricemia and/or hypercalciuria

            b. Usually occurs only if urine urate excretion >1 g/d

        5. Cystine (rare)

II. **Diagnostics**

    A. **History**

        1. Renal colic: severe flank pain to groin

        2. Hematuria: microscopic or gross

        3. Dysuria: frequency, urgency

        4. Factors predisposing to stone formation

            a. Estimation of daily fluid intake

            b. Recurrent UTIs

            c. Family history of stones and cause of stones

            d. Diet and medications

        5. Medical history

            a. Number of stones previously

            b. Treatments in past

            c. Gout

    B. **Examination**

        1. Abdominal and flank exam

        2. Signs of malignancy, inflammatory bowel, or skeletal disease

C. **Laboratory data**
  1. **Initial evaluation for single episode of renal calculi**
     a. Urinalysis (and culture if indicated)
     b. Electrolytes, creatinine and BUN
     c. Metabolites: calcium, magnesium, phosphate
     d. Uric acid
     e. Stone analysis: microscopy, x-ray crystallography
     f. Abdominal x-ray (flat plate)
     g. Intravenous urogram (IVU)
  2. **For selected patients with one episode of renal calculi**
     a. Urine cystine screening when stone not available
        for analysis
     b. PTH assay if patient hypercalcemic
     c. Renal tomograms if stones seen on plain or
        IVU films
  3. **For patients with history of 2 or more stones in a year or
     who have growing renal calculi**
     a. Routine laboratory, as above, plus the following
        i. Baseline 24-hr urine for volume, oxalate, citrate,
           pH, and creatinine
  4. **Monitor**
     a. If patient receiving treatment for recurrent stones
        i. Follow by 24-hr urine (as above) to see if treatment
           has had an effect on urine levels of stone forming
           substances
     b. Renal ultrasound is used by some practitioners to moni-
        tor for stones

III. **Management of Nonacute Calculi Disease**

A. **General approach**
  1. Increase fluid intake so as to increase urine output to
     >2 L/d
  2. Treat underlying disease(s), if present
B. **Preventive therapy** for recurrent stones
  1. **Calcium oxalate**
     a. Decrease calcium intake to <1 g/d
     b. Decrease salt intake
     c. Consider thiazide diuretic
     d. If patient hypocitraturic: vitamin C, up to 0.5–1 g/d
  2. **Stones with chronic UTI**
     a. Stone(s) must be completely removed (see below) for
        treatment to eradicate infection
     b. Antibiotic therapy is given for identified organisms
  3. **Uric acid stones**
     a. Alkalinize urine with bicarbonate or citrate
     b. Consider beginning allopurinol: 200–300 mg q.d.
        i. Dosage may be adjusted as determined by 24-hr
           urinary urate excretion
     c. Reduce dietary purines

IV. **Treatment of In Situ Stones**
  A. **General approach**
    1. Most urinary stones pass spontaneously; initial outpatient management is to ensure adequate fluid intake and pain control
    2. Open surgery is rarely used anymore
    3. Further treatment should be directed at renal or ureteric stones that are
      a. Symptomatic or potentially so
      b. Obstructive or potentially so
      c. Cause of infection
  B. If renal stone is **<5 mm in diameter and asymptomatic**
    1. No consensus on whether or not to treat
    2. Need to individualize therapy depending on patient characteristics
  C. **For renal stones >5 mm in diameter and needing treatment**
    1. Extracorporeal shock wave lithotripsy (ESWL)
      a. Is now used to clear approximately 60–90% of stones
      b. Best when kidney has single stone <2 cm in diameter
      c. With ureteral stones, ESWL can be used if location is in upper $^2/_3$ of ureter
      d. Contraindications
        i. Uncorrected bleeding diathesis
        ii. Inability of stone fragments to pass an obstruction
        iii. Pregnancy
        iv. Cystine stones
      e. Adverse effects
        i. Colic secondary to stone fragments
        ii. Acute vascular injury
        iii. Pancreatitis and GI bleeding (both rare)
        iv. Possible long-term renal damage (controversial)
  D. **For renal stones >2 cm or multiple stones,** combined therapy with percutaneous nephrolithotomy and ESWL is often used
  E. **Stones in lower $^1/_3$ of ureter** are usually removed by ureteroscopy
  F. **For infected stones of any size,** complete removal of stone and sterilization of urine must occur for cure

V. **Referral to Specialist for**
  A. Uncertainty of diagnosis or treatment
  B. Evaluation of and monitoring for recurrent renal stones
  C. Specialized management and procedures
  D. Complications due to calculi (e.g., obstruction)

References

1. National High Blood Pressure Education Program (NHBPEP): Review paper on complications of shock wave lithotripsy for urinary calculi. Am J Med 91:635–641, 1991.
2. NIH Consensus Conference: Prevention and Treatment of Kidney Stones. NIH. 7(1), March 30, 1988.

Rheumatic Fever

I. **General Principles**

   A. **Clinical and laboratory evidence** is used to discern evidence of major and minor Jones criteria

   B. Diagnosis requires
   1. 2 major **or** 1 major and 2 minor criteria
   2. **And** serological evidence of group A streptococcal infection
      a. **Note:** Group A skin infections do not cause acute rheumatic fever

   C. Lack of serologic evidence for streptococcal antibodies should cause a careful reevaluation of whether patient has rheumatic fever

   D. Rheumatic carditis usually involves the endocardium, myocardium, and pericardium and is almost always associated with valvulitis

II. **Diagnostics (Jones Criteria-Revised)**

   A. **Major manifestations**
   1. Carditis (in rheumatic fever, almost always associated with a murmur)
      a. Indications of carditis in a patient without previous rheumatic fever may be
         i. New murmur(s): mitral and/or aortic are usual
         ii. New cardiomegaly
         iii. Pericarditis
         iv. CHF without other apparent cause
      b. Indications of carditis in a patient with a history of previous rheumatic fever may be
         i. New murmur or significant change in old murmur
         ii. Increasing cardiomegaly
         iii. Pericarditis
   2. Polyarthritis in 2 or more joints (usually knees, ankles, wrists, and/or elbows) which are red, hot, tender, and swollen
   3. Chorea (Sydenham's) often occurs well after other manifestations
   4. Erythema marginatum
      a. Pink, nonpruritic annular lesion with pale center
      b. Mainly on trunk, never on face
      c. Can be induced by heat
   5. Subcutaneous nodules
      a. Firm, painless nodules often on extensor surfaces
      b. Also occur on occipital region and spinous processes

   B. **Minor manifestations**
   1. Prior history of rheumatic fever or rheumatic heart disease or evidence of prior rheumatic heart disease

2. Arthralgias cannot be used as minor criteria if polyarthritis present
3. Fever frequently is $>39°C$ ($102.2°F$) and is seen in early stages of rheumatic fever
4. Raised ESR or C-reactive protein (CRP) or leukocytosis
5. EKG with prolonged P-R interval

C. **Streptococcal antibody tests may be any (preferably 2) of**
1. ASO assay of >250 Todd units
2. Elevated or rising streptococcal antibody titers with serums drawn at 2–4 wk intervals
3. Throat culture (positive in about 25% of cases)

D. **Exceptions to Jones criteria**
1. Three instances when acute rheumatic fever should be considered without fulfilling Jones criteria and/or finding evidence of group A infection
   a. Recurrent rheumatic fever may occur with only a single major or several minor criteria (this needs evidence for recent group A infection)
   b. Indolent carditis without evidence of another known cause
   c. Chorea without evidence of another known cause

III. **Management**

A. Benzathine penicillin: 1.2 million units IM, single dose, even if cultures are negative
B. Codeine, high-dose aspirin, or corticosteroids for carditis
1. Discuss dosage with cardiologist, or ID specialist
2. Usual regimen is to continue 1 or combination of these for 2–3 wk after ESR or CRP is normal or nearly so, then taper drug(s)
C. Monitor success of therapy with periodic ESR or CRP
D. Following episode of rheumatic fever, most persons need daily antibiotic prophylaxis for at least 5 yr

IV. **Referral to Cardiologist or Infectious Disease Specialist for**

A. Uncertainty of diagnosis or treatment
B. Carditis
C. Follow-up of rheumatic heart disease

References

1. American Heart Association: Jones Criteria (revised) for guidance in the diagnosis of rheumatic fever. Circulation 69:204A, 1984.
2. American Heart Association: Guidelines for the Diagnosis of Rheumatic fever: Jones criteria, 1992 update. JAMA 268:2069–2073, 1992. (Note: the updated guidelines discuss only the diagnosis of the *initial* attack of acute rheumatic fever.)
3. Harrison's Principles of Internal Medicine, 12th ed. New York, McGraw-Hill, 1991, pp 933–938.

Rhinitis

I. **General Principles**

   A. Allergic rhinitis is a common atopic disorder and is an IgE-mediated hypersensitivity reaction to allergens, with typical symptoms including
   1. Sneezing
   2. Rhinorrhea
   3. Nasal congestion
   4. Itchiness of eyes and nose

   B. Other forms of rhinitis should be considered in a symptomatic individual
   1. **Vasomotor rhinitis**
      a. Symptoms similar to allergic rhinitis
      b. Allergen cannot be found
   2. **Perennial allergic rhinitis**
      a. Allergen and symptoms constant throughout year
      b. Often associated with nasal polyps and sinusitis
   3. **Reactive rhinitis** secondary to prolonged topical decongestant use

II. **Diagnostics**

   A. **History**
   1. Presence of above symptoms and relationship to seasons or to specific allergens
   2. Presence of asthma and/or sinusitis
   3. Previous nasal trauma
   4. Persistent use of topical decongestants
   5. Allergy to aspirin or other NSAIDs

   B. **Examination**
   1. Nasal anatomy for
      a. Deviated septum
      b. Nasal polyps
   2. Mouth examination for
      a. Masses or lesions
      b. Adenoid enlargement
   3. Neck examination for masses

   C. **Laboratory data**
   1. Diagnosis is usually based on clinical evaluation
   2. **Investigations may include**
      a. CBC and differential may show peripheral eosinophilia
      b. Nasal scrapings for eosinophils
      c. Skin testing
      d. IgE antibody tests (RAST and RIST)
         i. Radioallergosorbent tests (RAST) require specified allergens
         ii. Radioimmunosorbent tests (RIST)

III. **Management**
  A. **General approach**
    1. If a specific allergen can be identified, avoidance or reducing exposure is preferred
    2. Frequent allergens
      a. House mite and house dust
      b. Ragweed and other pollens
      c. Animal fur
      d. Molds and fungi
    3. For treatment of rhinitis, consider
      a. Antihistamines
      b. Topical steroids
      c. Oral decongestants and, when appropriate, stopping topical decongestants
  B. **Pharmacologic therapy**
    1. **Antihistamines** reduce sneezing, itching, and rhinorrhea but may cause drowsiness, especially in older patients
      a. Brompheniramine: 4 mg, every 4–6 hr and extended release 8 mg, every 8–12 hr
      b. Chlorpheniramine: 4 mg, every 4–6 hr
      c. Diphenhydramine: 25–50 mg, every 6–8 hr
      d. Tripolidine: 2.5 mg, every 4–6 hr
      e. If drowsiness is a problem, consider using a full dose at bedtime but a half dose, combined with an oral decongestant, during daytime, such as
        i. Actifed (triprolidine/pseudophedrine)
        ii. Drixoral (chlorpheniramine/pseudophedrine)
        iii. Allerest (chlorpheniramine/phenylpropanolamine)
      f. Newer antihistamines are less sedating but cost more
        i. Terfenadine (Seldane): 60 mg b.i.d.
        ii. Astemizole (Hismanal): 10 mg q.d., taken on an empty stomach
        iii. Avoid these drugs in patients taking medications that prolong QT intervals, or with electrolyte abnormalities, or with a history of ventricular arrhythmias
        iv. Do not exceed recommended doses
        v. Do not take astemizole or terfenadine concomitantly with erythromycin, ketoconazole or itraconazole
        vi. Avoid terfenadine and astemizole in patients with significant hepatic dysfunction
    2. **Decongestants**
      a. **Topical**
        i. Use for only 3–5 d and for the following reasons
          (a) To provide temporary relief from severe exacerbations of rhinitis
          (b) To allow topical steroids to be started
        ii. Selected examples and dosages
          (a) Phenylephrine: 1–2 sprays intranasally, q 4
          (b) Oxymetazoline (Afrin): 1–2 sprays, b.i.d.

       b. **Oral** (selected list)
         i. Pseudoephedrine HCL: 30–60 mg q.i.d.
           (a) Time-release capsule: 120 mg q 12 hr
         ii. Phenylpropanolamine: 20–25 mg q 4 hr
           (a) Extra release tabs: 75 mg q 12 hr
         iii. Considerations
           (a) Adverse effects of oral decongestants include insomnia and nervousness
           (b) Athletes who may need to undergo drug testing should not receive these drugs

  3. **Cromolyn sodium** (Nasalcrom)
    a. Used for allergic rhinitis and works best if used before expected exposures
    b. Also works well if begun prior to time of year when allergic exacerbations usually occur
    c. Dosages may be up to 2 inhalations, intranasally, 4–6 ×/d but some patients find lesser doses are effective

  4. **Intranasal topical steroids**
    a. Available preparations and dosages
      i. Flunisolide (Nasalide): 2 sprays b.i.d.
      ii. Beclomethasone (Beconase, Vancenase): spray or aqueous spray, 1 spray b.i.d.–q.i.d.
      iii. Triamcinolone (Nasacort): 2 sprays q.d.–b.i.d.
      iv. Dexamethasone (Decadron Turbinaire): 2 sprays b.i.d.–t.i.d.
    b. Taper starting doses to lowest effective level necessary to control symptoms (e.g., q.d. or q.o.d.)
    c. If patient has significant nasal irritation from drug after 1–2 wk, medication should be stopped
    d. Patients should not use higher than recommended doses
    e. Peak effect may take 1–2 weeks
    f. Duration of treatment usually depends on expected or known duration of symptoms (i.e., allergy season)

  5. **Immunotherapy**
    a. May work for individuals for whom specific allergens can be identified
    b. Refer to immunologist/allergist

IV. **Referral to ENT Specialist and/or Allergist for**
  A. Uncertainty of diagnosis or treatment
  B. Nasal anatomy abnormality
  C. Failure to respond to simple measures above
  D. Immunotherapy
  E. Suspicion of serious underlying disorder

References

1. Harrison's Principles of Internal Medicine, 12th ed. New York, McGraw-Hill, 1991, pp 1426–1428.
2. Med Lett 33:117, 1991.
3. Naclerio RW: Allergic rhinitis. N Engl J Med 325:860–869, 1991.

S

Sexually Transmitted Diseases

I. **General Principles**

  A. **High-risk groups**
   1. Sexually active persons < 25 y/o
   2. Persons with multiple sexual partners in the last 6 mo
   3. Persons with history of STD
   4. Prostitutes and those having sexual contacts with prostitutes
   5. Illicit drug users
   6. Inmates of detention centers

  B. **Routine health care for persons at risk for STD** should include the following
   1. Review of recent risk behaviors for STD
   2. Review of symptoms of STD
   3. Physical examination according to symptomatology
   4. Screening for asymptomatic infections in women
   5. Advice about
      a. Contraception, especially barrier methods
      b. Annual Pap smears

  C. **Patients infected with one STD should be evaluated for others**
   1. Patients with syphilis should be advised to get HIV test
   2. Persons with gonorrhea or chlamydia should be tested for syphilis; HIV testing should be discussed

II. **Diagnostics**

  A. **History**
   1. Prior diagnoses and treatments
   2. Duration, onset, and characteristics of STD symptoms
   3. Sexual behavior: number of partners, type of sexual activity
   4. Systemic complaints: rash, joint pain, fever, malaise
   5. Allergies to penicillin or other drugs

  B. **Examination**
   1. Skin examination for rash
   2. Throat examination if history of orogenital contact
   3. Abdominal palpation for tenderness, masses
   4. Evaluation of genitalia and urethra in men
   5. Pelvic exam: speculum and digital exam in women
   6. Rectal exam in selected cases
   7. Lymph nodes for adenopathy

  C. **Laboratory data for symptomatic persons**
   1. **Women**
      a. Cervical cultures for *N. gonorrhoeae* and *C. trachomatis*
      b. Gram stain and/or KOH preparation

    c. Wet mount of vaginal secretions

    d. Pregnancy test (important in drug choice and in further counseling and management)

  2. **Men**

    a. Urethral cultures for *N. gonorrhoeae* and *C. trachomatis*

  3. **When STD is found,** both genders should be considered for syphilis serology (VDRL or RPR)

D. **Laboratory data for selected situations**

  1. **For genital ulcerations**

    a. Culture or antigen test for HSV

    b. Serologic tests for syphilis (VDRL or RPR)

    c. Culture for *H. ducreyi*

    d. Dark-field exam for spirochetes

  2. **For mucopurulent cervicitis** (MPC)

    a. Gram stain and culture for gonorrhea

    b. Test for chlamydia

    c. Wet mount for trichomonas

  3. **For epididymitis in young man** (< 35 y/o)

    a. Urinalysis and culture

    b. Consider urethral culture

  4. **For asymptomatic pregnant women**

    a. Initial prenatal screening should include

      i. Cultures for chlamydia and gonorrhea

      ii. Syphilis serology (VDRL or RPF)

    b. If in high-risk category, repeat screening in 3rd trimester

    c. HIV testing should be considered in women with risk factors or in women who wish to be tested

III. **Management: General Approach**

A. Prevention is **always** appropriate

  1. Education about sexual behaviors such as

    a. Abstinence

    b. Contraceptives, including condoms and spermicides for optimal HIV protection for a sexually active person

  2. Informing sexual partner(s) when STD diagnosed

  3. Notification of known or presumed diagnosis to health authorities for gonorrhea, syphilis, chlamydia, trichomonas, chancroid, lymphogranuloma

B. **Treatment for selected symptoms/signs**

  1. **For mucopurulent cervicitis**

    a. Treat as per test results or, if unavailable, treat empirically for

      i. *N. gonorrhoeae*

      ii. *C. trachomatis*

      iii. See below for regimens

    b. Evaluate sexual partners for STD

2. **For epididymitis in young man** (<35 y/o)
   a. Consider empiric treatment for
      i. *N. gonorrhoeae*
      ii. *C. trachomatis*
   b. Evaluate sex partners for STD if above pathogens found

IV. **Chancroid *(Haemophilus ducreyi)***
   A. **General presentation**
      1. Painful genital ulcer
      2. Painful inguinal lymphadenopathy (50% of patients)
   B. **Treatment is either one of**
      1. Erythromycin: 500 mg PO q.i.d. × 7 d
      2. Ceftriaxone: 250 mg IM, single dose
   C. **Alternative treatments include any one of**
      1. Trimethoprim/sulfamethoxazole: 160/800 mg b.i.d. × 7 d
      2. Amoxicillin (500 mg) + clavulanic acid (Augmentin) × 7 d
      3. Ciprofloxacin: 500 mg PO b.i.d. × 3 d
   D. **Monitoring treatment**
      1. If no improvement within 7 d, review
         a. Compliance
         b. Coexistence of another STD
         c. HIV risk factors
         d. Antibiotic resistance
      2. FNA can be done if lymphadenopathy persists
   E. **Sexual contacts**
      1. All partners within 10 d prior to development of symptoms in patient should be evaluated and treated, whether symptomatic or not

V. **Syphilis *(Treponema pallidum)***
   A. **General presentation**
      1. **Primary stage**
         a. May be entirely absent
         b. Characterized by chancre (painless papule with an indurated edge)
            i. Can appear on penis, labia, cervix, anus, or mouth 10–90 d after exposure
            ii. Heals within 2–6 wk, leaving no scar
      2. **Secondary stage**
         a. Maculopapular rash involving any part of body 6 wk–6 mo after exposure
         b. Relapses of secondary stage may occur without treatment
      3. **Latent stage**
         a. Clinically silent
         b. Early latent is defined as <1 yr
         c. Late latent is >1 yr
      4. **Tertiary stage**
         a. Cardiovascular in 10–20% of untreated cases
         b. Neurosyphilis in 4–6% of untreated cases
         c. Gummas

B. **Diagnostics**
   1. **For ulcers or tissue sample**
      a. Dark-field examinations
      b. Direct fluorescent antibody tests
   2. **Serum serology**
      a. VDRL or RPR with quantification by dilutional titers
         i. 1:8 is considered positive
         ii. 1:4 is possibly positive
      b. Laboratory should verify a positive test by using disease-specific serologies
   3. **Indications for CSF serology**
      a. Neurologic abnormalities
      b. Failure of previous treatment (see below)
      c. Patient has had syphilis for >1 yr
      d. Patient has had syphilis for unknown duration

C. **Treatment**
   1. **Early syphilis**
      a. Definition
         i. Primary or secondary disease
         ii. Early latent disease
      b. Drugs
         i. Benzathine penicillin (PCN) G: 2.4 MU IM × 1
         ii. For penicillin-allergic patients any of:
            (a) Doxycycline: 100 mg PO b.i.d. × 14 d
            (b) Tetracycline: 500 mg PO q.i.d. × 14 d
            (c) Erythromycin: 500 mg PO q.i.d. × 14 d
   2. **Late disease**
      a. Definition
         i. >1 yr duration
         ii. Cardiovascular syphilis
         iii. Gummas
         iv. Late latent
      b. Drugs
         i. Penicillin (benzathine) G: 2.4 MU IM weekly for 3 wk
         ii. For penicillin-allergic patients either of
            (a) Doxycycline: 100 mg PO b.i.d. × 30 d
            (b) Tetracycline: 500 mg PO q.i.d. × 30 d
   3. **Neurosyphilis** (outpatient treatment)
      a. Definition (CSF examination)
         i. VDRL of CSF is usually positive, but may be negative in some cases of neurosyphilis
         ii. Leukocyte count >5 WBC/mm^3
         iii. Total protein >40 mg/100 ml
      b. Drugs
         i. Aqueous procaine PCN G: 2.4 MU IM q.d. × 10–14 d
            and
         ii. Probenecid: 500 mg PO q.i.d. × 10–14 d

D. **Monitoring**
   1. Reevaluate at 3 and 6 mo with serologies
   2. For neurosyphilis
      a. Check CSF at 3 and 6 mo
      b. Many practitioners admit for IV penicillin rather than give outpatient treatment as above
   3. Treatment failures need CSF examination and are defined as a VDRL or RPR titer that has not declined
      a. Fourfold by 3 mo with primary or secondary syphilis
      or
      b. Fourfold by 6 mo with early latent syphilis
   4. Encourage patient to consider an HIV test
E. **Sexual contacts**
   1. Partners should be evaluated and treated appropriately
F. **Special consideration**
   1. HIV-infected persons with positive syphilis serology
      • See chapter on "HIV and Syphilis" for details

VI. **Lymphogranuloma Venereum *(Chlamydia trachomatis)***

A. **General presentation**
   1. Genital and/or anorectal ulcer with lymphadenopathy
   2. Often confused with chancroid
B. **Diagnostics**
   1. As per any genital or anorectal ulcer
C. **Treatment**
   1. Doxycycline: 100 mg PO b.i.d. × 21 d
D. **Alternative treatments** (any of)
   1. Tetracycline: 500 mg PO q.i.d. × 21 d
   2. Erythromycin: 500 mg PO q.i.d. × 21 d
   3. Sulfisoxazole: 500 mg PO q.i.d. × 21 d

VII. **Genital and Anal Herpes (Herpes Simplex Virus)**

A. **General presentation**
   1. Painful, indurated ulcer, often with surrounding small papules
   2. Infection occurs when uninfected mucous membrane is exposed to symptomatic partner
   3. HSV may infrequently be spread by asymptomatic carrier
B. **Diagnostics**
   1. As per genital or anorectal ulcer
C. **Treatment**
   1. **General approach**
      a. **As no cure exists,** therapy aims to reduce symptomatic recurrences and reduce duration of episodes
      b. **Recurrent episodes are treated if severe**
         i. Start treatment as early as prodromal symptoms, if possible
         or
         ii. Within 48 hr of ulcer appearance

    c. **Suppressive therapy**
       i. Reduces recurrences by about 75%
       ii. Considered if patient has > 6 episodes/yr
       iii. Discontinue after 1 yr to review recurrence rate
    d. **Education about herpes**
       i. Discuss natural history of disease
       ii. Advise abstention from contact from prodromal symptoms until lesion fully healed
       iii. Advise condom use during sexual contact
       iv. Explain risk of neonatal infections
       v. Pregnant women should inform obstetrician of diagnosis

2. **For first clinical episode of genital HSV**
    a. Initiate therapy as soon as possible after onset
    b. Acyclovir: 200 mg PO 5 ×/d (q 4 hr) for 7–10 d or until clinical resolution occurs
    c. **Severe first episodes** may need inpatient admission for treatment with IV acyclovir

3. **For first clinical episode of herpes proctitis**
    a. Acyclovir: 400 mg PO 5 ×/d for 10 d or until clinical resolution occurs

4. **For treatment of recurrences in severe disease**
    a. Begin treatment within 2 d, preferably when prodromal symptoms are noted
       i. Acyclovir: 200 mg PO 5 × d **or** 800 mg PO b.i.d. × 5 d

5. **Suppressive therapy for chronic prophylaxis**
    a. Indicated for use up to 1 yr
       i. Acyclovir: 200 mg PO 2–5 ×/d
       or
       ii. Acyclovir: 400 mg PO b.i.d.

6. **Special circumstances**
    a. **Pregnancy**
       i. Acyclovir is used only for life-threatening HSV infections (e.g., encephalitis)
    b. **HIV and AIDS**
       i. Infected persons may need higher doses for treatment and suppression
       ii. Try regimen(s) as given above
         (a) If needed, refer or consult for resistant disease

VIII. Gonococcal Infections *(Neisseria gonorrhoeae)*

A. **General approach**
1. Strains found in the U.S. include penicillin- and tetracycline-resistant organisms
2. Chlamydial infection occurs frequently in persons with gonorrhea and is treated concomitantly
3. Cultures should be done for all suspected cases of gonococcal disease for antibiotic susceptibility

   4. Treatment is given (once cultures are sent) for
      a. Presumed infection
      b. Sexual contacts of persons with documented infection
   5. Encourage patients to have HIV test
B. **Diagnostics**
   1. Cultures are sent for suspected infections and may include rectum, pharynx, urethra, endocervical, or joint aspirates
   2. Syphilis serology should be requested for all those with presumed gonococcal infection
   3. Notification should be sent to health authorities
C. **Treatment**
   1. **For uncomplicated gonococcal infection**
      a. Ceftriaxone: 250 mg IM, single dose
         and
      b. Doxycycline: 100 mg PO b.i.d. × 7 d
   2. **Alternative treatments** (selected listing)
      a. Alternatives to ceftriaxone (any one of)
         i. Ofloxacin: 400 mg PO, single dose
         ii. Spectinomycin: 2 g IM, single dose
         iii. Ciprofloxacin: 500 mg PO, single dose
         iv. Norfloxacin: 800 mg PO, single dose
         v. Cefotaxime: 1 g IM, single dose
      b. Alternatives to doxycycline (either of)
         i. Tetracycline: 500 mg q.i.d. × 7 d
         ii. Erythromycin: base 500 mg q.i.d. × 7 d
   3. **Special circumstances**
      a. *T. pallidum* is not susceptible to spectinomycin or quinolones, so patients receiving these drugs should have syphilis serology after 1 mo for treatment of gonococcal infections
      b. Documented penicillin-susceptible gonococcus may be treated with
         i. Amoxicillin: 3 g PO, single dose
            and
         ii. Probenecid: 1 g, single dose
            and
         iii. Doxycycline as above (for *C. trachomatis*)
      c. **For pharyngeal gonococcal infection**
         i. Treatment is either one of
            (a) Ceftriaxone: 250 mg IM, single dose
            (b) Ciprofloxacin: 500 mg PO, single dose
         ii. Reculture 4–7 d after treatment
      d. **Pregnant women and nursing mothers**
         i. For treatment of gonococcal infection
            (a) Ceftriaxone as above
               or
               Spectinomycin: 2 g IM, single dose, for PCN-allergic patients
               and
            (b) Erythromycin stearate: 500 mg PO q.i.d. × 7 d

    ii. Reculture pregnant women 4–7 d after treatment

    iii. Do not use quinolones and tetracyclines

  e. **For disseminated infection,** admit for IV antibiotics

D. **Monitoring**

  1. **For persons treated with ceftriaxone/doxycycline**

    a. Must return if symptoms persist after treatment

    b. Consider reculture 1–2 mo after treatment

  2. Persons treated with antibiotics other than ceftriaxone/doxycycline need follow-up cultures 4–7 d after regimen completed

E. **Sexual partners**

  1. Exposure to gonorrhea within 4 wk necessitates examination, cultures, and treatment as given above

IX. **Chlamydial Infections**

A. **General approach**

  1. Chlamydia may cause asymptomatic infection

  2. Screening is recommended for high-risk groups

  3. Chlamydia is a frequent cause of PID

B. **Diagnostics**

  1. Abdominal and pelvic examination for signs of PID

  2. Diagnosis either by culture or nonculture methods

  3. Send cultures for *N. gonorrhoeae* as well

C. **For treatment of uncomplicated urethral, endocervical, or rectal infection** when gonorrhea is not found

  1. Use one of

    a. Doxycycline: 100 mg PO b.i.d. × 7 d

    b. Erythromycin stearate: 500 mg PO q.i.d. × 7 d

  2. Alternative treatments may be one of

    a. Sulfisoxazole: 500 mg PO q.i.d. × 10 d

    b. Erythromycin ethylsuccinate: 800 mg PO q.i.d. × 7 d

D. **Special considerations in pregnancy**

  1. Treat with erythromycins as listed above

  2. Erythromycin estolate, sulfisoxazole, and doxycycline are contraindicated

E. **Monitoring**

  1. Repeat cultures are not necessary after treatment

F. **Sexual partners**

  1. Recent sexual contacts should receive examination, cultures, and treatment as per above regimen

X. **Nongonococcal Urethritis (NGU)—*C. trachomatis, Ureaplasma urealyticum, Trichomonas vaginalis,* HSV**

A. **General approach**

  1. Diagnosed by Gram stain demonstrating abundant PMN without intracellular gram-negative diplococci

  2. *C. trachomatis* has been implicated as the cause of NGU in 50% of cases

B. **Diagnostics**
1. Urethral or cervical cultures (including chlamydial) and Gram stain
2. Wet mount for trichomonas
3. If ulceration present, evaluate as per above (p. 234)

C. **Treatment consists of one of**
1. Doxycycline: 100 mg PO b.i.d. × 7 d
   or
2. Tetracycline: 500 mg PO q.i.d. × 7 d
3. Alternative treatments include one of
   a. Erythromycin stearate: 500 mg PO q.i.d. × 7 d
   b. Erythromycin ethylsuccinate: 800 mg PO q.i.d. × 7 d
   c. Erythromycin ethylsuccinate: 400 mg PO q.i.d. × 14 d

D. **Monitoring**
1. If NGU does not respond, consider reinfection or noncompliance with therapy
2. If noncompliance is the presumable cause, repeat above therapeutic regimen
3. If compliance is likely, repeat therapy with alternative regimen
4. If urethritis continues after treatment(s), refer to or consult with STD specialist

E. **Sexual partners**
1. For partners of men, evaluate and treat as per clinical findings

XI. **Vaginosis and Vaginal Diseases**

A. *Trichomonas vaginalis*
1. Almost always sexually transmitted
2. **Diagnostics**
   a. Wet mount with direct microscopic visualization
   b. **Or** by culture
3. Treatment is either of
   a. Metronidazole: 2 g PO, single dose
   b. Metronidazole: 500 mg PO b.i.d. × 7 d
4. **Monitoring**
   a. If either of above regimens fails, treat (again) with metronidazole: 500 mg PO b.i.d. × 7d
   b. If still no response, use metronidazole: 2 g PO q.d. × 3–5 d
   c. If still no response, check susceptibility to metronidazole and refer to or consult with STD specialist
5. **Sexual partners**
   a. Treat with either single-dose or 7-d therapeutic regimen
6. **Special considerations in pregnancy**
   a. Metronidazole should not be used in first trimester and should be avoided, if possible, during all of pregnancy
   b. For severe symptoms, consider metronidazole, 2 g, single dose, given after first trimester

B. **Bacterial *(Gardnerella)* vaginosis**
1. Usually caused by alterations in normal vaginal flora
2. **Diagnostics**
   a. Vaginal discharge
   b. pH > 4.5
   c. Amine odor test
   d. Clue cells on Gram stain or wet mount
3. **Treatment**
   a. Asymptomatic infection has no consensus on whether to treat; treatment is optional
   b. Symptomatic infection with metronidazole: 500 mg PO b.i.d. × 7 d
4. **Sexual partners**
   a. No evaluation or treatment necessary

C. **Candida vaginitis**
1. **General approach**
   a. Vaginal candidiasis (yeast infection or moniliasis) usually presents as genital irritation and itching and may be associated with a heavy, sometimes thick and cheesy, white discharge
   b. Although not an STD, it can be passed between sexual partners
   c. For women with frequent infections, partners should be evaluated for a source (e.g., ballanitis)
2. **Diagnostics**
   a. Usually by visual inspection and/or finding yeast on KOH preparation
3. **Treatment** may include such antifungals as
   a. Miconazole: 2% cream, intravaginally q.d. × 7 d
   b. Miconazole suppositories: 100–200 mg intravaginally q.d. × 3 d
   c. Clotrimazole (Gyne-Lotrimin): 500 mg intravaginally, single dose, or 100 mg intravaginally q.d. × 7 d
4. **Monitoring**
   a. Not necessary
   b. Women with frequent infections should have their partner(s) assessed for ballanitis

XII. **Condylomata Accuminata (Genital Warts)**

A. **General approach**
1. Caused by a group of different human papillomaviruses (HPV)
2. Incubation period ranges from 1–6 mo
3. Infection may cause clinical warts or be subclinical
4. No treatment completely eliminates HPV infection; recurrence rates are high for all therapies

B. **Diagnostics**
1. Warts on the penis and on the labia and introitus are easily seen on examination

    2. Colposcopy is often used to evaluate vaginal and cervical lesions

C. **Treatment**

    1. Patient-applied treatment is available in the form of Podofilox (podophyllotoxin): 0.5% solution applied by applicator b.i.d. × 3 d

       a. After 4-d interval treatment may be repeated if needed

       b. This 7-d cycle may be repeated up to 4 ×

       c. Patient should use no more than 0.5 ml of Podofilox per day and should use the smallest amount necessary to coat the warts

       d. This drug is for external genital warts only

    2. Other treatments

       a. Physician-applied podophyllin solutions

       b. Laser or cryosurgery

       c. Electric cauterization

D. **Sexual contacts**

    1. Partners may be treated as per symptoms

    2. Patients engaging in sexual contact should be instructed to use barrier methods to help reduce risk of infection to partners

E. **Special consideration**

    1. Women with history of exposure should have yearly cervical smears

XIII. **Ectoparasitic Infections**

A. **Lice** *(Pediculosis pubis)*

    1. Lice or eggs are often found at hair-skin junction

    2. **Treatment** may be one of

       a. Lindane cream and lotion: rub into skin and hair, leave in place for 8–12 hr, then wash thoroughly

       b. Lindane 1% shampoo: scrub hair for 4 min, then rinse off completely

       c. Permethrin 1% creme (for **head** lice only): wash and rinse after 10 min

    3. **Monitoring**

       a. Review after 1 wk if symptoms persist

       b. Repeat treatment if lice or eggs found

    4. **Sexual partners**

       a. Treat contacts concurrently with patient

    5. **Special considerations**

       a. Lindane is not used for pregnant or lactating women

       b. Machine-wash and/or dry contaminated clothing and linens

B. **Scabies** *(Sarcoptes scabiei)*

    1. **General approach**

       a. Scabies mite causes progressive, itchy, papular, and/or eczematous rash, often with burrows

       b. Itching is often worse at night

2. **Diagnostics**
    a. Glass slide with cover slip of scrapings of papule
    b. Microscopic exam of slide after KOH preparation
3. **Treatment**
    a. Lindane 1% applied from neck to toes, then washed off completely after 8 hr
    b. Alternative treatment: Crotamiton 10%
        i. Apply from neck to toes, repeat 24 hr later, and wash off completely 48 hr after last application
        ii. Keep away from eyes and mouth
4. **Monitoring**
    a. If no improvement in 1 wk, repeat treatment with one of above regimens
5. **Sexual partners and close (household) contacts**
    a. Treated as above
6. **Special considerations**
    a. Lindane should not be used for pregnant or lactating women
    b. After treatment, itching may continue for 1–3 wk
    c. Machine-wash (hot) and dry contaminated clothes, linens

XIV. **Referral to STD Specialist or Gynecologist for**

A. Uncertainty of diagnosis or treatment
B. Persistent STD or symptoms
C. Treatment failures
D. Monitoring of syphilis status
E. Evaluation of high-risk persons
F. Evaluation and monitoring of pregnant and/or breast-feeding women

References

1. Centers for Disease Control: Sexually transmitted diseases: Treatment guidelines. MMWR 38(S-8), 1989.
2. Drugs for sexually transmitted diseases. Med Lett 33:119-121, 1991.
3. Podofilox for genital warts. Med Lett 33:118, 1991.

Sinusitis

I. **Definition**

Sinusitis refers to infection or inflammation of any of the sinuses

II. **General Principles**

A. **Sinusitis may involve**
    1. Maxillary sinus
    2. Ethmoid sinus
    3. Sphenoid sinus
    4. Frontal sinus

B. Acute sinusitis does not generally need an extensive evaluation before treatment but further investigation is suggested if
  1. >3 or 4 recurrences/yr
  2. Sinus problems interfere with working or leisure activities
  3. Poor response to medical therapy
  4. Sinus disease exacerbates other medical problems (e.g., asthma, COPD)
  5. Anatomic abnormality is noted (e.g., deviated septum)
  6. Serious disease is suspected (e.g., carcinoma of the nasopharynx)

III. Diagnostics

A. **History**
  1. Duration of symptoms
  2. Facial pain, headaches, watery eyes
  3. Type of discharge from nose
  4. Exposure to possible allergens
  5. Seasonal changes and red, itchy eyes (which may indicate allergy-mediated sinusitis)

B. **Examination**
  1. Palpation of sinuses for tenderness
  2. Examination of mouth and throat, ear, nasal passages
  3. Evaluation of neck for masses, lymphadenopathy
  4. Auscultation of chest

C. **Laboratory data**
  1. Diagnosis of acute sinusitis is usually by clinical evaluation
  2. For evaluation of chronic symptoms, consider
     a. **Plain sinus x-rays** (usually sufficient)
        i. Maxillary sinus mucosal thickening of >6 mm is associated with bacterial infection
        ii. Fluid level(s) in sinuses
     b. **4-cut CT scan of sinuses**
        i. Request coronal sections of sinus(es) with bone window settings
        ii. Accurate method of diagnosis and may be less expensive than series of radiographs
     c. For fiberoptic rhinoscopy with or without biopsy, refer to ENT specialist
     d. Allergy testing (skin) in selected patients with
        i. History of seasonal sinus complaints
        ii. Worsening symptoms with environmental antigens associated with worsening of asthma

IV. Management

A. **For acute, uncomplicated sinusitis**
  1. Consider simple measures such as
     a. Nasal decongestant for 2–3 d
     b. Steam and/or saline spray inhalations

    2. Antibiotic course of 14–21 d if bacterial infection suspected
      a. Amoxicillin: 500 mg t.i.d.
      b. Trimethoprim/sulfamethoxazole: 160/800 mg b.i.d.
      c. Doxycycline: 100 mg b.i.d.

B. For chronic or recurrent sinusitis
1. Antibiotic therapy as above, for 3–4 wk
2. Moderate to maximum doses of nasal decongestant (tablets) for 1 mo (e.g., pseudoephedrine, 120 mg, or guaifenesin, 600 mg b.i.d.)
3. Corticosteroid nasal inhaler b.i.d. for 1 mo (e.g., beclomethasone nasal spray, 2 inhalations b.i.d.)
4. Steam and saline inhalations for 30 d
5. Consider work-up if no response or if evaluation/symptoms indicate possible underlying disorder
    a. Nasal polyp or deviated septum
    b. Sinus or nasopharynx tumor
    c. Bloody discharge

C. For suspected allergy-mediated sinus problems
1. Refer if possible to allergist or specialist for skin testing
2. Can temporize with
    a. Antihistamine of choice
    b. Nasal corticosteroid
    c. Oral decongestants

V. Referral to Ear, Nose, and Throat Specialist for

A. Uncertainty of diagnosis or treatment
B. Suspected anatomic abnormalities (deviated septum)
C. Suspected obstructive disease (e.g., polyp, CA)
D. Differentiation from other diseases that may present as chronic sinusitis (e.g., ear or throat pathology)
E. Failure of medical therapy

Reference

Druce HM, Slavin RG: Sinusitis: A critical need for further study. J Allergy Clin Immunol 88:675–677, 1991.

Syncope

I. Definition

Syncope is a sudden and temporary loss of consciousness and postural tone, with spontaneous recovery

II. General Principles

A. Wide arrays of diagnostic technologies are usually unnecessary and not cost-effective or goal-oriented

B. No matter what the work-up, 40–50% of cases are not diagnosed
  1. Cardiac causes are found in about 10–40% of cases, depending on study cohort
  2. A normal EKG indicates very low likelihood of arrhythmias or sudden death

III. **Diagnostics**
  A. **History**
    1. Memory of event and just prior to event
      a. Rapidity of onset
      b. Presence of premonitory or warning event
      c. Vasovagal symptoms
    2. Chronology and number of event(s)
    3. Observation of episode by witness
    4. Incontinence or tongue-biting
    5. Postural symptoms
    6. Detailed drug history and timing of drugs
    7. Whether associated with micturition, cough, swallowing
    8. Alcohol and substance use
    9. Medications, including timing (e.g., synergistic effects with each other)
  B. **Examination**
    1. Blood pressure measurements in both arms
      a. > 20 mmHg difference in BP between arms is suggestive of subclavian steal syndrome
    2. Orthostatic changes of **BP** and **pulse** with associated postural symptoms: supine and then after 3 min of standing (or with legs over the bed if patient unable to stand)
    3. Mental status and neurologic exam
    4. Detailed **cardiac exam** for
      a. Pulse character and regularity
      b. Valvular disease
      c. CHF
    5. Abdominal exam for masses, AAA
    6. Stool hemoccult test
  C. **Laboratory data**
    1. **Initial investigations**
      a. CBC and differential (anemia, infection)
      b. Electrolytes, especially K+
      c. Glucose (hypoglycemia)
      d. Cr/BUN for renal disease
      e. Magnesium, phosphorus, calcium for episodes thought secondary to arrhythmia
      f. EKG is abnormal in about 50%
        i. Most abnormalities are LVH, old MI, fascicular blocks
  D. **Further investigations**
    1. **Drug and/or alcohol levels:** if abuse suspected

2. **Holter monitor** (24–72 hr)
   a. Especially if patient has
      i. Underlying cardiac disease
      ii. EKG is abnormal
      iii. Symptoms of arrhythmia
   b. In general, holter monitor is rarely helpful in patients younger than 60 y/o with normal EKG
3. **Echocardiogram** with evidence of
   a. Valvular disease
   b. Reduced cardiac output (including HOCM, CHF)
   c. Evidence of an old infarct on EKG
   d. Exertional syncope, especially in a young adult
4. **CT and/or EEG**
   a. In patients who have
      i. Evidence or a history of focal neurological deficit
      ii. Possible seizure disorder
   b. They are almost never helpful in other cases
5. **Transtelephonic monitoring and intermittent loop recorders**
   a. Helpful in near-syncope, dizziness, and pacemaker failure
   b. Patient must be aware enough to dial telephone once symptoms have begun
6. **Exercise testing** should be considered if
   a. History suggests ischemic-induced arrhythmia or symptoms
   b. Syncope occurs during exercise
7. **Carotid massage** should be considered for carotid sinus hypersensitivity
   a. Which occurs in less than 1% of patients
   b. Patient must be on a monitor with cardiac resuscitation kit nearby when this is done
   c. Contraindicated if patient has carotid bruit
8. **Upright tilt testing** with or without isoproterenol infusion is occasionally used when testing for neurally mediated syncope (vasovagal syndrome)
9. **Signal average EKGs**
   a. Detects low amplitude signals (late potentials) in terminal portion of QRS complex
   b. Sometimes used as screening for VT
   c. Usefulness has not been fully defined, as yet
10. **Electrophysiological study (EPS) should be considered if**
    a. Potentially dangerous arrythmia is noted on EKG or on ambulatory monitoring
    b. Recurrent undiagnosed syncope, especially in patients with severe cardiac disease
    c. Patient has Wolff-Parkinson-White syndrome

IV. **Management**
   A. Treatment is governed by clinical findings and relevant investigations

B. Many cases of syncope are not found to have an obvious cause and reassurance to patient and family is important

C. In recurrent syncope of unknown cause patient may need fairly extensive evaluation and referral for one or more of the above sophisticated tests

D. Postural syncope may respond to
1. Changing the timing of hypotension-inducing drugs or changing to a different drug or drug formulation (e.g., long-acting tablet)
2. Use of support stockings
3. Increasing fluid volume or decreasing diuretic therapy, when appropriate
4 Moderate doses of prostaglandin inhibitors (NSAIDs)

V. **Referral May Be Considered for**

A. Uncertainty of diagnosis or management
B. For suspected or documented cardiac disease
C. For significant postural hypotension not responsive to simple measures
D. Suspected or documented neurologic disease or seizure disorder

References

1. Kapoor WN: Diagnostic evaluation of syncope. Am J Med 90:91–106, 1991.
2. Manolis AS, Linzer M, Salem D, Estes NAM: Syncope: Current diagnostic evaluation and management. Ann Intern Med 112:850–863, 1990.

T

Thyroid Disorders

I. **General Principles**
   A. Screening tests for thyroid disorders for asymptomatic individuals are generally unwarranted
   B. They should be considered for adults at risk for developing thyroid disorders, including those who
      1. Have a strong family history of thyroid disease
      2. ≥65 y/o
      3. Have autoimmune disease(s)
      4. Are postpartum women, 4–8 wk after delivery
   C. Thyroid tests are often used when evaluating
      1. Arrhythmias such as atrial fibrillation
      2. Depression and other psychiatric disorders
      3. Persons with a history of thyroid disease or radiation to the neck
      4. Persons with clinically suspected thyroid disease
      5. Persons with goiter
      6. Nonspecific symptoms that may be due to thyroid disease (such as fatigue, significant weight changes)
   D. Avoid thyroid imaging studies in asymptomatic patients who do not have palpable thyroid nodules
   E. Men >60 y/o with thyroid nodules are at high risk for having thyroid cancer

II. **Diagnostics**
   A. **General approach**
      1. Diagnosis attempts to document **clinical** thyroid status: hypo-, eu-, or hyperthyroid
      2. Presence or absence of palpable abnormalities of the thyroid gland
   B. **History**
      1. Evaluation of changes in
         a. Weight and appetite
         b. Personality and/or emotional lability (including depressive symptoms)
         c. Sensitivity to cold or warm (climatic) temperatures
         d. Changes in bowel habit
         e. Sleep
         f. Menstrual cycle
         g. Strength and general energy levels
         h. Texture and loss of hair
         i. Cardiovascular and respiratory systems (shortness of breath, palpitations, or angina)
         j. Prior neck irradiation

    k. Family history of thyroid disease(s) or multiple endocrine neoplasias (MEN)

  2. Presence of enlargement of thyroid gland

    a. Onset and duration of abnormality

    b. Local symptoms (dysphagia, hoarseness, or pain)

    c. Previous history of nodules

C. **Examination**

  1. General: skin and hair texture

  2. Head and eyes for facial and ocular abnormalities

    a. Periorbital edema

    b. Facial puffiness

    c. Exophthalmos

  3. Neck palpation: presence or absence of goiter

  4. Cardiovascular: resting pulse rate and pulse character

  5. Neurologic: general status and reflexes

  6. Limbs: tremor, pretibial myxedema

D. **Laboratory data**

  1. Recommended **initial tests** when thyroid disorder suspected

    a. TSH: sensitive test (sTSH) preferred

    b. Free thyroxine level: FT4

      i. FTI may be substituted if FT4 unavailable

  2. **Laboratory tests for selected situations**

    a. If **nodular or diffuse goiter** is noted, request initial tests above and thyroid microsomal antibodies or thyroglobulin antibodies

    b. If the patient has clinical evidence of **Graves' disease**, request initial tests as above and thyroid microsomal antibodies or thyroglobulin antibodies

    c. If patient has clinical evidence of **Hashimoto's or postpartum thyroiditis**, request initial tests as above and thyroid microsomal antibodies or thyroglobulin antibodies

    d. **Further investigations**

      i. If testing indicates that patient may have pituitary-induced hyper- or hypothyroidism, refer to or consult with endocrinologist

      ii. If patient is euthyroid, without goiter, and has abnormal TSH and normal FT4 (or FTI), follow patient clinically and consider requesting thyroid microsomal antibodies or thyroglobulin antibodies

      iii. If patient has enlarged thyroid and test-documented hyperthyroidism, a nuclear scan with iodine-123 differentiates

        (a) Diffuse toxic goiter (Graves' disease)

        (b) Toxic nodular goiter

        (c) Thyroiditis (low thyroid uptake)

      iv. **If patient has enlarged thyroid and laboratory-documented euthyroidism**

        (a) For solitary or dominant nodule, perform a fine needle aspiration (FNA)

          (i) If FNA indicates follicular neoplasm, request radioiodine scan to differentiate functional (hot) nodule from a nonfunctional (cold) nodule

      (b) For palpable multinodular goiter, consider a pertechnetate scan to differentiate functional (hot) areas and nonfunctional (cold) areas

      (c) Refer cold nodules for FNA

3. Alternative methodologies

    a. Some practitioners suggest that thyroid nodules should undergo ultrasound evaluation in addition to nuclear scanning prior to FNA

      i. Usually not cost-effective

      ii. FNA indicates when nodule is cystic and gives information on cell cytology when nodule is solid

    b. Some practitioners recommend that all nodules, whether hot or cold, be evaluated by FNA

      i. In this case, prior nuclear scanning is not usually done

III. Management

A. General approach for selected entities

1. For solitary nodule

    a. Management depends on result of FNA

      i. Benign nodules are either observed or may be treated with T4 suppression

      ii. Malignant nodules are surgically removed

    b. Nonfunctioning nodules >2 cm are usually surgically excised but this may depend on biopsy result

      i. Refer to endocrinologist for details

    c. Nodules that are suspicious for cancer (rapid growth, very firm, associated lymphadenopathy should be surgically removed regardless of tissue diagnosis)

2. Hashimoto's thyroiditis is treated once patient is clinically hypothyroid by replacement with L-thyroxine (T4)

3. For Graves' disease and toxic nodular goiter, treatment is undertaken in consultation with endocrinologist

4. For subclinical hyper- or hypothyroidism

    a. Physicians may elect to clinically observe with periodic monitoring of FT4 (or FTI) and (s)TSH

    b. Subclinical hypothyroidism is often treated, however

B. Monitoring

1. For replacement therapy with L-thyroxine

    a. Monitor with TSH or (s)TSH

      i. Keep TSH within normal range

      ii. If dosage of T4 changed, recheck TSH at 6–8 wk

      iii. Some practitioners use FT4 as well as TSH because FT4 can give an **approximation** of response to new or newly-changed L-thyroxine therapy

b. **Caution:** in patients with coronary artery disease, replacement therapy should begin at low dose and increase gradually to avoid worsening ischemia/angina
c. For suppression therapy with L-thyroxine, monitoring TSH with or without FT4 should be undertaken in consultation with an endocrinologist because extent of suppression depends on type of disorder (e.g., thyroid cancer, benign nodule)
2. After treatment for hyperthyroidism, monitor by periodic
    a. Clinical evaluation
    b. FT4 (or FTI) and TSH

IV. **Referral**
A. After initial evaluation of thyroid disorder, further diagnostic investigations and initial management are usually done in consultation with or by referral to an endocrinologist or specialist in thyroid disease

References

1. American Thyroid Association: Guidelines for use of laboratory tests in thyroid disorders. JAMA 263:1529–1532, 1990.
2. Bayer MF: Effective laboratory evaluation of thyroid status. Med Clin North Am 75:1–21, 1991.
3. Greenspan FS: The problem of the nodular goiter. Med Clin North Am 75:195–209, 1991.
4. Thyroid cancer in thyroid nodules: Finding a needle in the haystack (editorial). Am J Med 93:359–362, 1992.

Tuberculosis

I. **Definition**
A. Tuberculosis is caused by airborne mycobacterium, including
    1. *M. tuberculosis*
    2. *M. bovis*
    3. *M. africanum*

II. **General Principles**
A. The following persons have increased risk for acquiring TB and should be screened for infection every 6–24 mo
    1. Close contacts of person known or suspected to have TB
    2. Foreign-born persons from countries with high TB prevalence (e.g., Africa, Asia, Latin America)
    3. Persons from lower socioeconomic groups
    4. Residents of long-term care or prison facilities
    5. Persons with silicosis, jejunoileal bypass, gastrectomy
    6. Chronic disorders: end-stage renal disease, substance abuse
    7. Immunosuppression: diabetes, HIV, medications

8. Weight loss of 10% or more below ideal body weight
9. Leukemias, lymphomas and reticuloendothelial malignancies
10. Persons with old healed TB on CXR examination
B. Preventive treatment is given to asymptomatic persons with a positive PPD but with no evidence of TB on CXR
C. Skin tests such as Tine and Purified Protein Derivative (PPD) are used for screening and diagnosis

III. Diagnostics

A. History
1. Respiratory symptoms of cough (with or without sputum), chest pain, hemoptysis
2. Systemic symptoms: weight loss, fevers, night sweats
3. Disseminated manifestations: bone pain, lymphadenitis, cognitive changes, headaches
4. Medication and medical history, especially
   a. Previous TB treatment(s)
   b. Medical or other risk factors for TB
   c. Prior use of and/or previous reactions to isoniazid
   d. Acute or chronic liver disease
   e. Medications and alcohol history
   f. Presence of peripheral neuropathy or diabetes
5. Pregnant

B. Examination
1. Respiratory exam
2. Systematic review for disseminated disease

C. Laboratory data
1. For PPD, induration in mm is read at 48–72 hr after placement
2. Positive PPDs for specified risk groups are defined as
   a. **PPD ≥5 mm is considered positive in**
      i. Persons having close contacts with active TB and no known PPD reaction in past
      ii. HIV-infected individuals (see also chapter on "HIV and Tuberculosis")
      iii. History of old TB by CXR
   b. **PPD ≥10 mm is considered positive with**
      i. Recent converters (defined as)
         • ≥10 mm increase within 2 yr, if patient is <35 y/o
         • ≥15 mm increase within 2 yr, if patient is ≥35 y/o
      ii. Intravenous drug user with negative HIV test
      iii. Medical conditions predisposing to TB (see above)
      iv. Persons under 35 y/o who are from
         (a) Medically underserved populations
         (b) Residents in care facilities or prisons
         (c) Immigrants from countries with high prevalence

c. **PPD ≥15 mm is considered positive in**
  i. Persons under 35 y/o with no risk factors
d. **No preventive therapy is required if**
  i. PPD >10 mm in persons >35 y/o and without any of above risk factors or symptoms of disease
  ii. Person has had previous positive PPD because of vaccination with BCG and is without risk factors or symptoms
3. If PPD is positive, request chest x-ray (PA)
  a. If CXR suspicious for TB infection
    i. Send 3 morning sputums for stains/culture
    ii. If patient unable to provide sputum, consider induction or referral for bronchoscopy
4. **If antitubercular medications are to be started,** request
  a. CBC and platelets
  b. Liver function tests: SGOT, SGPT, bilirubins, alkaline phosphatase
  c. Serum creatinine and BUN
  d. Uric acid (for pyrazinamide therapy)
  e. Visual examination (for ethambutol therapy)
5. **Further investigations** may include any of
  a. Urinalysis for sterile pyuria
  b. Imaging studies (e.g., x-ray) for suspected bony disease or disseminated TB
  c. Lumbar puncture: for suspected TB meningitis

IV. **Management**

A. **For preventive therapy** when PPD is positive with no evidence of pulmonary or extrapulmonary tuberculosis
  1. Isoniazid 300 mg PO q.d. × 6–12 mo
    or
  2. Isoniazid 15 mg/kg (to 900 mg) twice wk × 6–12 mo
    a. Monitor monthly for symptoms of hepatitis, abdominal pain, and peripheral parasthesias
    b. Check transaminases if symptoms indicate hepatic toxicity
      i. In persons >35 y/o, check SGOT or SGPT periodically as these patients have an increased risk for liver toxicity
      ii. Consider stopping isoniazid if either transaminase becomes >3–5× normal range
  3. Pyridoxine 50 mg q.d. should be given in persons with
    a. Evidence of peripheral neuropathy
    b. HIV infection
    c. Diabetes, uremia, alcoholism, malnutrition
    d. Pregnancy
    e. Seizure disorders
  4. **Special considerations**
    a. Use 12 mo of isoniazid if person is HIV-infected or has CXR with evidence of old nonactive TB

    b. If isoniazid-resistant tuberculosis suspected or proven, use rifampin with or without ethambutol (standard doses given below)

    c. If patient unable to take isoniazid, treat as per isoniazid-resistant TB

    d. Women who are pregnant should have preventive therapy after birth unless there is strong evidence of recent infection or they are symptomatic

       i. Treatment should be discussed with an ID specialist

B. Management for pulmonary or disseminated tuberculosis

    1. Consider respiratory isolation, until after treatment begun, for patients with active pulmonary TB

    2. General approaches for treatment

      a. 6-mo regimen with

        i. 2 mo of isoniazid, rifampin, and pyrazinamide, then 4 mo of isoniazid and rifampin

          (a) Addition of ethambutol when isoniazid resistance is suspected

      b. 9-mo regimen of isoniazid and rifampin

        i. Add ethambutol if isoniazid resistance suspected

      c. Twice weekly therapy may, in some cases, be started after 1–2 mo of daily therapy (discuss with specialist)

    3. For details regarding therapy for resistant TB, consult local ID, pulmonary, or other specialist

    4. Instruct patients on possible adverse reactions and monitor, as listed above, if symptoms develop

    5. Follow patients at least monthly during treatment

    6. Compliance is essential to treatment

    7. **Specific drugs (first-line therapy)**

      a. **Isoniazid:** tablets of 100 mg, 300 mg

        i. Daily dose: 5 mg/kg PO or IM (up to 300 mg)

        ii. Twice weekly dose: 15 mg/kg (up to 900 mg)

        iii. Drug interaction

          (a) Dilantin and INH together can increase the serum concentration of both

      b. **Rifampin:** capsules of 150 mg, 300 mg

        i. Daily dose: 10 mg/kg PO (up to 600 mg)

        ii. Twice weekly dose: 10 mg/kg (up to 600 mg)

        iii. Major side effect is orange secretions and urine

        iv. Drug interactions include inducing hepatic microsomal enzymes

      c. **Pyrazinamide:** 500 mg tablets

        i. Daily dose: 15–30 mg/kg PO (up to 2 g)

        ii. Twice weekly dose: 50–70 mg/kg

        iii. Major adverse reactions

          (a) Hepatotoxicity

          (b) Hyperuricemia

          (c) Arthralgias

       (d) Skin rash
       (e) Gastrointestinal upset
    d. **Streptomycin:** vials of 1 g and 4 g
      i. Daily dose: 15 mg/kg IM (up to 1 g)
      ii. Twice weekly dose: 25–30 mg/kg IM
      iii. Major adverse reactions
       (a) Ototoxicity
       (b) Nephrotoxicity
      iv. If possible, avoid in patients >60 y/o
    e. **Ethambutol:** tablets of 100 mg, 400 mg
      i. Daily dose: 15–25 mg/kg/d PO (up to 2.5 g)
      ii. Twice weekly dose: 50 mg/kg
      iii. Major adverse reactions
       (a) Decreased red-green color discrimination
       (b) Decreased visual acuity
      iv. Baseline visual acuity and color discrimination should be checked
8. **Monitoring** for patients with active TB
    a. **For patients with AFB in sputum,** monitor with monthly stains and culture of sputum until no further AFB is found
    b. If AFB found at 3 mo after beginning treatment
      i. Request a drug susceptibility test
      ii. Consider giving therapy under supervision if non-compliance with drug treatment is suspected
    c. If resistant mycobacterium found, ensure treatment includes at least 2 drugs to which the organisms are susceptible
    d. At completion of drug regimen, repeat sputum culture and stains
    e. **For patients with abnormal chest x-ray at baseline**
      i. Repeat CXR within 2–3 mo of starting therapy
      ii. If no improvement after 3 mo
       (a) Consider an alternative diagnosis
       (b) TB is old and not active
    f. For patients on isoniazid, monitor transaminases as listed above
    g. To ensure adequate therapy, close follow-up should be provided for patients who have had only 6 mo of treatment or for immunosuppressed patients who have had 9 mo of treatment
    h. Patients should be instructed to return if they develop cough, fever, or weight loss
    i. **Treatment failures** are defined as persons with AFB in sputum at 5 mo or with relapse of disease after therapy is finished
      i. These patients should be reevaluated by an ID specialist
9. **Special considerations in pregnancy**
    a. Do not use streptomycin or pyrazinamide

V. Referral to ID or Pulmonary Specialist for

A. Uncertain of diagnostic or therapeutic protocols
B. Further diagnostics
C. Follow-up and monitoring
D. Treatment failures
E. Complications of pulmonary or disseminated TB
F. Pregnant patients

VI. Notification

A. Tuberculosis is a reportable disease
B. Check public health codes in your area for specifics

References

1. American Thoracic Society/Centers for Disease Control: Treatment of tuberculosis and tuberculosis infection in adults and children. Am Rev Respir Dis 134:355–363, 1986.
2. Centers for Disease Control: Screening for tuberculosis and tuberculosis infection in high-risk populations: Recommendations of the Advisory Committee for Elimination of Tuberculosis. MMWR 39:1–12, 1990.

Tumor Markers

I. General Principles

A. No marker is infallible; its usefulness depends on
   1. Sensitivity of the test(s)
   2. Specificity of the test(s)
   3. Prevalence in the population tested
B. In an asymptomatic population the use of known markers identifies far more false positives than true positives
   1. Most markers are not always cancer-specific
C. All evaluations have financial and psychological costs as well as morbidity and mortality associated with the work-up
D. **Markers in regular use and their associated cancers**
   1. Alpha-fetoprotein (AFP): testicular, hepatocellular
   2. Human chorionic gonadotropin (beta-HCG): testicular, gestational trophoblastic
   3. Lactate dehydrogenase (LDH, LDH-1): testicular
   4. Carcinoembryonic antigen (CEA): colorectal
   5. Prostatic acid phosphatase (PAP): prostate
   6. Prostate-specific antigen (PSA): prostate
   7. CA 125: ovary
E. Markers are used in tandem with clinical evaluation, not alone

II. Diagnostics

A. **History and examination are used to establish**
   1. Whether marker is necessary

2. What the pretest risk of disease is
3. Potential complicating factors in interpreting marker

B. **Specific diseases and markers**
  1. **Prostate**
    a. **Prostatic acid phosphatase** (PAP)
       i. Elevation detects 85–95% of patients with metastatic disease
       ii. It does not detect early prostatic CA and is not generally useful in the work-up of prostatism
    b. **Prostate-specific antigen** (PSA)
       i. May be elevated in benign prostatic hyperplasia
       ii. Levels >10 ng/ml indicate greater likelihood of prostate cancer
       iii. Rising PSA levels after therapy for CA usually indicate recurrence
       iv. PSA response tends to reflect response to treatment of prostate cancer
       v. Useful to monitor patients who have undergone any form of treatment for prostatic cancer, especially radical prostatectomy
       vi. It is not an effective screening tool for prostatic cancer
          • For further details see the chapter on "Prostatism"
  2. **Colorectal**
    a. **CEA can be present in other conditions,** including carcinomas of breast or lung
       i. It is not an accurate screening test in the asymptomatic population
       ii. It has low sensitivity and specificity in early CA of colon
       iii. Steadily rising levels over 1 mo after resection usually indicate recurrence
    b. **Recommendations for use of CEA**
       i. To monitor for recurrences of colon cancer in persons who have been treated for such
       ii. It is not used in screening asymptomatic populations
  3. **Hepatocellular**
    a. **AFP is useful as screening test in highly selected populations**
       i. In hepatitis B-positive patients with chronic active hepatitis or cirrhosis, accuracy of detecting hepatocellular cancer is
          (a) Sensitivity: 65%
          (b) Specificity: 98%
       ii. Estimate of prevalence of hepatocellular cancer in persons with chronic hepatitis B liver disease (data from China) is 2800 in 100,000

b. **Recommendations for use**
   i. For patients with cirrhosis or CAH
      (a) AFP levels every 3–4 mo
      (b) Ultrasound every 4–6 mo
4. **Ovarian**
   a. **CA-125 may be elevated in**
      i. Benign or malignant ovarian disease
      ii. Endometriosis
      iii. Salpingitis
      iv. Uterine myoma
      v. Pregnancy (1st trimester)
   b. **Disease prevalence and CA-125 test dynamics**
      i. General population prevalence is 30 in 100,000 (1 in 3,300 women)
         (a) Test has sensitivity of 80%, specificity of 99%
         (b) Thus only about 2.5% (1 in 40 women) of those with positive tests will actually have ovarian cancer
      ii. In women with a pelvic mass, prevalence of ovarian cancer is about 10% (1 in 10)
         (a) CA-125 for this group has sensitivity of 80–87%, specificity of 78–88%
         (b) Thus an elevated test in a woman with a pelvic mass gives a 40% (2 in 5) chance of cancer
         (c) A negative test gives a 2.5% (1 in 40) chance of finding cancer
   c. **Recommendations for use**
      i. CA-125 is not currently used for screening asymptomatic women
      ii. It may assist in helping evaluate a pelvic mass
      iii. A normal CA-125 does not exclude malignancy
      iv. It may be useful in monitoring women with known ovarian CA who have had an elevated CA-125
      v. If ovarian cancer is suspected, request ultrasound and refer

References

1. Bates SE: Review: Clinical applications of tumor markers. Ann Intern Med 115:623–638, 1991.
2. Di Bisceglie AM, Rustgi VK, Hoofnagle JH, et al: Hepatocellular carcinoma. Ann Intern Med 108:390–401, 1988.
3. Fletcher RH: Carcinoembryonic antigen. Ann Intern Med 104:66–73, 1986.

U

Urinary Incontinence

I. **Definition**

Incontinence refers to the **involuntary loss of urine**

II. **General Principles**

A. Incontinence affects all age groups, including 15–30% of those >65 y/o and up to ½ of nursing home residents
B. Prevalence in women is about twice that in men
C. Drug effects and physical or mental disabilities are frequent causes that can often be modified easily
D. **Incontinence may be generally categorized as**
   1. **Stress incontinence** refers to urinary leakage when laughing, coughing, walking and is often associated with
      a. Multiparity
      b. Weakness of pelvic floor muscles
   2. **Urge incontinence** is the inability to inhibit loss once the urge to void is sensed and is often due to
      a. Local factors such as cystitis, atrophic urethritis or vaginitis, bladder cancer
      b. Neurologic dysfunction such as demyelinating disease or stroke
   3. **Overflow incontinence** is due to overdistention of bladder with large postvoid residual, often because of mechanical/functional obstruction such as
      a. Prostatic hypertrophy, urethral stricture or fecal impaction
      b. Drugs (e.g., anticholinergics, antihistamines, tricyclic antidepressants, antipsychotics)
      c. Spinal lesions
   4. **Reflex incontinence** is caused by uninhibited bladder contractions
   5. **Functional incontinence** is the inability to reach the toilet
      a. Immobility or severe cognitive deficit
      b. Drugs (e.g., benzodiazepines, alcohol, antipsychotics)
   6. **Multifactorial causes of incontinence** often occur in the frail elderly

III. **Diagnostics**

A. **History**
   1. Age of onset
   2. Type(s) of incontinence (as above)
   3. Precipitants and timing of incontinence

4. Fluid intake (timing, types of beverages)
5. Frequency of incontinence: per day, week, or month
6. Presence of dysuria, urinary frequency, hesitancy, straining, urgency
7. Presence of prostatic symptoms in men
8. Volume
   a. Drops
   b. Small (wets underwear)
   c. Large (wets clothes or bedding)
9. Alterations in bowel habit and/or sexual function
10. General medical (arthritis, diabetes mellitus)
11. Parity in women
12. Surgical history (pelvic or GU)
13. Neuropsychiatric (dementia, stroke, neurologic impairment)
14. Functional status
    a. Mobility, dexterity
    b. Mental state
    c. Activities of daily living

B. **Examination**
   1. General mental status
   2. Neurologic assessment
   3. Abdominal examination for masses and estimation of postvoid residual (PVR)
   4. Digital rectal examination for masses, prostatic size
   5. Pelvic for masses, cystocele, prolapse
   6. Genital examination for abnormalities of foreskin or glans penis
   7. Functional capability, including mobility and dexterity
   8. Provocative stress testing (leakage of urine is watched for while patient coughs vigorously)

C. **Laboratory data**
   1. **Usual initial investigations**
      a. Serum electrolytes, glucose, creatinine and BUN
      b. Urinalysis and culture
      c. Postvoid residual
         i. Normal: <50 ml
         ii. Abnormal: ≥200 ml
         iii. Inconclusive: 50–199 ml
   2. **Further investigation**
      a. Urine cytology for patients with hematuria or for those with irritative symptoms but without evidence of a UTI
      b. **Imaging studies** (most are ordered by specialists)
         i. For pelvic or abdominal mass, consider ultrasound scan or CT scan
         ii. For suspected overflow incontinence
            (a) Cystometrogram (pressure flow study)
            (b) Cystoscopy
            (c) Videourodynamics

      iii. For suspected stress incontinence
         (a) Stress cystourethrogram
         (b) Dynamic profilometry
      iv. If hematuria found or for evaluation of possible bladder cancer, consider
         (a) Intravenous urogram (IVU)
         (b) Cystourethroscopy

IV. Management

A. General approach
1. Discontinue potentially offending drug(s)
2. Diuretics may worsen any type of incontinence
3. Treat urinary tract infections
4. If mobility decreased, consider use of bedside urinal or commode and scheduled toileting
5. Surgical management should be considered for
   a. Significant urethrocele or other prolapse
   b. Mechanical obstruction (e.g., BPH)
   c. Intrinsic sphincter dysfunction
   d. Detrussor instability refractory to medical treatment

B. For stress or urge incontinence
1. **Behavioral techniques**
   a. Pelvic floor (Kegel) exercises can benefit men and women
   b. Biofeedback may improve symptoms in up to 50% of patients
   c. Bladder training to void at regular, progressively longer intervals

C. For stress incontinence
1. Useful drugs include
   a. Alpha-adrenergic agents such as phenylpropanalomine: 25–75 mg (in sustained-release form) PO b.i.d.
   b. Estrogen therapy when atrophic urethritis/vaginitis is considered as a cause of the stress incontinence
     • See chapter on "Hormone Replacement Therapy" for details
   c. Impipramine: 10–25 mg q.d.–t.i.d.

D. For urge incontinence
1. Useful drugs include
   a. Oxybutynin (Ditropan): 5 mg b.i.d.–t.i.d.
     i. Maximum is 20 mg/d
   b. Propantheline: 7.5 mg–30 mg t.i.d.–5 ×/d, taken on an empty stomach
   c. Tricyclic antidepressant agents such as impipramine (10–25 mg q.d.–t.i.d.) and doxepin (10–25 mg, q.d.–t.i.d.)
   d. Estrogen therapy (local or oral), when incontinence is thought due to atrophic vaginitis/urethritis
     • See chapter on "Hormone Replacement Therapy" for details

E. **For patients who are incontinent despite treatment**
1. Absorbent pads or underwear
2. Catheters: indwelling or condom type for men

V. **Referral for**

A. Uncertainty of diagnosis or management
B. Failure of medical therapy
C. Lower GU or pelvic surgery/irradiation within past 6 mo
D. Frequently recurrent or relapsing symptomatic UTI
E. Severe symptoms of prostatism
F. Stress incontinence in a man
G. Severe stress incontinence in a woman
H. Symptomatic pelvic prolapse
I. Suspicion of prostatic carcinoma
J. Postvoid residual >200 ml
K. Microhematuria in the absence of bacteriuria and pyuria
L. Failure to respond to medical treatment
M. Need for sophisticated diagnostic imaging tests

References

1. National Institutes of Health: Consensus conference: Urinary incontinence in adults. JAMA 261:2685–2690, 1989.
2. Ouslander J, Leach G, Staskin D, et al: Prospective evaluation of an assessment strategy for geriatric urinary incontinence. J Am Geriatr Soc 37:715–724, 1989.
3. Urinary Incontinence Guideline Panel: Urinary Incontinence in Adults and Quick Reference Guide for Clinicians. AHCPR Publication Nos. 92-0038 and 92-0041. Rockville, MD, Agency for Health Care Policy Research (AHCPR), Public Health Service, U.S. Department of Health and Human Services, 1992.

Urinary Tract Infection

I. **Definition**

Urinary tract infection (UTI) refers to a spectrum of entities of symptomatic or, in some cases, asymptomatic invasion of organisms into the lower and/or upper urinary tract

II. **General Principles**

A. **UTI commonly occurs in women (10–20% lifetime prevalence)**
1. Most (90%) UTIs (in women) are caused by
   a. *E. coli*
   b. *Enterobacter*
   c. *S. saprophyticus*
   d. *Enterococcus*
2. Elderly women are not usually treated for asymptomatic bacteriuria

3. Elderly men are not usually treated for asymptomatic bacteriuria unless the patient is
   a. Immunodeficient
   b. Going to have genitourinary instrumentation
   c. Known to have significant urinary tract abnormality
4. Women with multiple recurrent UTI may benefit from prophylactic antibiotics (see below for details)

B. **Type of UTI** helps to determine treatment regimen and follow-up
1. **Uncomplicated lower UTI** is acute cystitis with irritative symptoms, including dysuria, burning, frequency, suprapubic pain
2. **Complicated lower UTI** is subacute pyelonephritis with symptoms of acute cystitis and one or more complicating factors listed below
3. **Uncomplicated upper UTI** is mild acute pyelonephritis with flank tenderness, minimal toxicity (temperature <102 F), stable vital signs, ability to care for self, and tolerance for fluids
4. **Complicated upper UTI** is moderate to severe acute pyelonephritis in which the patient is toxic, does not tolerate fluids, and has high temperature, unstable or potentially unstable vital signs, elevated white cell count, and/or is unable to care for self

C. The following should be treated as complications of lower UTI (subacute pyelonephritis)
1. Pregnancy
2. Indwelling catheter, GU tract abnormality, recent GU instrumentation, or hospital acquired infection
3. Lower socioeconomic status, including homelessness
4. Recurrent UTI after recent treatment or >3 UTIs in past year
5. UTI before age 12
6. Duration of symptoms >7 d prior to receiving therapy
7. Immunodepressant syndromes, including diabetes, drugs, alcohol abuse, HIV
8. Recent treatment with antibiotics for any reason

III. **Diagnostics**

A. **History**
1. Presence of UTI symptoms
   a. Dysuria
   b. Hematuria
   c. Urgency
   d. Incontinence
   e. Suprapubic or pelvic pain
2. Presence of risk factors listed above
3. Systemic symptoms: fever, sweats, nausea, vomiting
4. Penile discharge
5. Vaginitis (chlamydial UTI or atrophic urethritis)

B. **Examination**
  1. Vital signs for temperature, pulse and blood pressure
  2. Abdominal examination for
     a. Suprapubic tenderness (specific for cystitis)
     b. Renal mass
     c. Flank: costovertebral angle (CVA) tenderness
     d. Inguinal lymphadenopathy
  3. In men, genital/scrotal examination for
     a. Testicular tenderness or masses
     b. Urethral discharge
     c. Penile lesions or glans inflammation
  4. If clinical suspicion (i.e., vaginal discharge, symptoms of prostatism) warrants
     a. Pelvic exam for signs of vaginitis
     b. Prostate exam in men
C. **Laboratory data**
  1. **Usual initial investigation:** urinalysis
     a. Hematuria, pyuria, or bacteriuria
     b. Gram stain
     c. Positive leukocyte esterase
  2. **Investigations when clinically indicated**
     a. Cultures
        i. Should be sent when **subacute or acute pyelonephritis** is suspected in any patient or for any type of UTI if patient is **male**
        ii. Diagnostic if >1000 colonies/ml of a specific organism
     b. CBC with differential if clinical suspicion is of systemic infection
     c. Electrolytes, Cr and BUN should be sent if
        i. Renal insufficiency suspected
        ii. Renal mass is palpated
        iii. Patient is male
     d. Urethral or cervical/vaginal studies with suspicion of STD
        • See chapter on "STDs" for details
     e. Imaging studies
        i. **Intravenous urogram (IVU)** considered for
           (a) Pyelonephritis with
               (i) Renal colic symptoms
               (ii) Failure of medical therapy after 3 d
               (iii) Suspected intrarenal abscess
           (b) Suspected underlying urinary tract abnormality or obstruction
               (i) Pyelonephritis in a man
               (ii) Recurrent (≥3) UTIs per yr in a woman
               (iii) Renal mass
               (iv) Associated renal parenchymal disease
        ii. **Ultrasound scan** indications are similar to IVU

IV. **Management**
  A. **General approach**
    1. **Acute uncomplicated cystitis** is treated with antibiotic of choice for 3–5 d (or single-dose therapy) in women, but for 7–10 d in men
    2. **Acute complicated cystitis** (subacute pyelonephritis) is treated with antibiotic of choice for 7–10 d
    3. **Acute uncomplicated (mild) pyelonephritis** is treated with antibiotic of choice for 14 d
    4. **Acute complicated pyelonephritis** is treated with hospitalization and IV antibiotics
  B. **Antibiotic therapy**
    1. **Inexpensive,** with good coverage
      a. Doxycycline: 100 mg b.i.d.
      b. Tetracycline: 500 mg q.i.d.
      c. Trimethoprim: 100 mg b.i.d.
      d. Trimethoprim/sulfamethoxazole: 160/800 mg b.i.d.
      e. Amoxicillin: 500 mg t.i.d.
      f. Cephalexin: 500 mg q.i.d.
    2. **More expensive,** with good coverage
      a. Ciprofloxacin: 250 mg b.i.d.
      b. Norfloxacin: 400 mg b.i.d.
      c. Amoxicillin/clavulanate: 500 mg b.i.d.
      d. Newer cephalosporins
  C. **Special considerations**
    1. Prophylaxis for women with recurrent UTIs is considered for 2–3 symptomatic UTIs within 6 mo or >3 symptomatic UTIs within 1 yr
      a. Trial of antibiotic therapy, usually for 6 mo
      b. Some women may prefer postcoital antibiotic prophylaxis if UTIs are temporally related to coitus
      c. For continuous prophylaxis consider any of
        i. Nitrofurantoin: 50 mg q.d.–b.i.d.
        ii. Trimethoprim/sulfamethoxazole: 40/200–80/400 q.d. or 3 ×/wk
        iii. Trimethoprim: 100 mg q.d.
        iv. Cephalexin: 125–250 mg q.d.
      d. For postcoital prophylaxis
        i. Nitrofurantoin: 50–100 mg
        ii. Trimethoprim/sulfamethoxazole: 80/400
        iii. Cephalexin: 250 mg q.d.
    2. **Pregnant women**
      a. Are treated for **asymptomatic or symptomatic** bacteriuria to reduce risk of premature delivery and further urinary tract disease
      b. Can be treated with
        i. Amoxicillin: 500 mg t.i.d. or ampicillin 500 mg q.i.d.

        ii. Cephalexin: 500 mg q.i.d.

        iii. Erythromycin: 500 mg q.i.d.

   c. Should not receive

        i. Ciprofloxacin, norfloxacin at any time

        ii. Tetracyclines at any time

        iii. Sulfonamides in 3rd trimester

3. **Men with UTI** (summary)

   a. Assess possibility of prostatitis, epididymitis

   b. Request urine culture

   c. Check Cr, BUN for renal dysfunction

   d. Treat with antibiotic of choice for 7–10 d with coverage for *C. trachomatis* and *N. gonorrhoeae* in young men with epididymitis

   e. Obtain posttreatment culture

   f. Not all men need further studies after a single episode of uncomplicated cystitis

      i. Different age groups may, however, need assessment for underlying urinary tract abnormalities

        (a) In the elderly population, consider evaluation for BPH

        (b) In the younger population, consider evaluation for congenital abnormalities with studies such as IVU or ultrasound

   g. Recurrent or refractory UTIs need evaluation by urologist

D. **Monitoring**

1. Posttherapy cultures at 1–2 wk are needed for

   a. Persisting symptoms

   b. Persons with complicating factors (listed above)

   c. Acute pyelonephritis: uncomplicated or complicated

   d. Men with a UTI

2. Posttherapy cultures are not necessary for resolved acute cystitis in women

V. **Referrals to Urologist Should Be Considered for**

A. Acute complicated cystitis or pyelonephritis

B. Uncertainty of diagnosis or treatment

C. Abnormality on imaging study

D. UTI in a man

References

1. Hooten TM, Stamm WE: Management of acute uncomplicated urinary tract infections in adults. Med Clin North Am 75:351–352, 1991.
2. Johnson JR, Stamm WE: Urinary tract infections in women: Diagnosis and treatment. Ann Intern Med 111:906–917, 1989.
3. Lipsky BA: Urinary tract infections in men: Epidemiology, pathophysiology, diagnosis, and treatment. Ann Intern Med 110:138–150, 1989.

W

Weight Loss

I. Definition

  A. The definition of significant involuntary weight loss is arbitrary but practical guidelines may include any of
    1. >5% of body weight over 6 mo
    2. Change in clothing size
    3. Objective quantification by previous weight in medical record
    4. Supportive evidence as given by an observer

II. General Principles

  A. Up to 50% of persons complaining of weight loss have not lost weight
  B. Causes of weight loss may be unidentifiable in up to $^1/_3$ of persons with that complaint
  C. **Common causes of involuntary weight loss**
    1. Change in diet
    2. Cancer: lung, lymphoma, GI tract, metastatic disease
    3. Gastrointestinal diseases
    4. Chronic diseases, CHF, COPD
    5. Alcohol abuse
    6. Infectious diseases: TB, HIV
    7. Psychiatric illness: depression, dementia
    8. Medications

III. Diagnostics

  A. **History**
    1. Amount and duration of weight loss
    2. Change in appetite
    3. Diet and nutrition history
    4. Smoking and alcohol history
    5. Gastrointestinal complaints: nausea, vomiting, dysphagia, diarrhea
    6. Respiratory complaints: cough, shortness of breath, chest pain
    7. Presence and location of pain
    8. HIV risk factors
    9. Systemic symptoms: fatigue, malaise, sweats, fevers, chills
    10. Ability to perform activities of daily living
      a. Cooking and preparing foods
      b. Buying groceries

B. **Examination**
   1. General mental state and minimental status exam
   2. Head and neck examination
   3. Presence of lymphadenopathy
   4. Respiratory examination
   5. Abdominal and genital/pelvic examination for masses
   6. Rectal examination for hemoccult test
C. **Laboratory data**
   1. **Routine** (for patients whose history does not indicate a specific cause for the weight loss)
      a. CBC and differential
      b. Electrolytes and Cr, BUN
      c. Liver function tests
      d. Thyroid tests: FT4 and TSH
      e. Urinalysis
      f. CXR
   2. **For selected patients**
      a. HIV test
      b. For those with primarily GI complaints, consider
         i. UGI series
         ii. Ba enema
      c. For a positive hemoccult
         • See chapter on "Colorectal Cancer"
      d. PPD or tine test

IV. **Management**
   A. Management is governed by results of evaluation
   B. For patients whose diagnosis remains elusive, closely follow over 6 mo and monitor and quantify weight at each visit
   C. Depression should always be a consideration
      1. Evaluate patients for vegetative signs
      2. Discuss recent life events and changes

Reference

Marton K, Sox H: Involuntary weight loss: Diagnostic and prognostic significance. Ann Intern Med 95:568–574, 1981.

PART VII
MEDICAL DECISION-MAKING

Probability Theory and Clinical Decisions

I. **Definition of Probability Theory**

   A. Probability theory was developed from the work of Thomas Bayes, an 18th-century English clergyman

   B. Bayes' theorem allows clinicians to estimate the probability (0–100%) that a person has a disease, given a positive or negative test or evaluation

II. **General Principles**

   A. **The following are needed for decision-making**
   1. The clinician's initial estimate (from 0–100%) that a patient has a specific disease **before** the patient undergoes a test or evaluation (the **pretest estimate**)
   2. An estimate on **how good a test/evaluation is** in finding the disease **(sensitivity)** and how good it is in determining when the disease is not there **(specificity)**
   3. A way to calculate the estimate (from 0–100%) that a patient has a disease **after** the test result has been taken into account (the **posttest probability**)
   4. A way to interpret the probabilities (the **diagnostic decision**)

   B. **Almost any test/evaluation can be so used,** including
   1. All or part of the history (e.g., hot, red, painful big toe)
   2. All or part of the examination (e.g., Murphy's sign)
   3. A screening tool (e.g., CAGE questions)
   4. The laboratory investigations (e.g., CEA for colon cancer)
   5. The imaging studies (e.g., an ultrasound for cholecystitis)

   C. **But** the sensitivity and specificity of the test/evaluation must be known

III. **Testing a Test or an Evaluation**

   A. Determination of the capability of a test is represented by
   1. **Sensitivity:** an estimate (0–100%) of how often a positive test picks up actual disease (the true positive rate)

$$= \frac{\text{true positives (TP)}}{\text{true positives (TP)} + \text{false negatives (FN)}}$$

2. **Specificity:** an estimate (0–100%) of how often a negative test means absence of disease (the true negative rate)

$$= \frac{\text{true negatives (TN)}}{\text{true negatives (TN)} + \text{false positives (FP)}}$$

3. The sensitivity and specificity of a test are determined by comparing a given test's results for a specific population of patients to actual pathology (autopsy) or, more commonly, to a "gold standard" test
   a. This is frequently represented as a **2 × 2 table**

	Disease Present	Disease Absent
Test result positive	TP	FP
Test result negative	FN	TN

   b. Sensitivity and specificity can be derived from the table
   c. The **predictive values** for negative and positive tests can also be calculated

B. **Predictive value:** the probability that a test result is correct
   1. **Positive predictive value**

   $$= \frac{\text{TP}}{\text{All Positives}} = \frac{\text{TP}}{\text{TP} + \text{FP}}$$

   2. **Negative predictive value**

   $$= \frac{\text{TN}}{\text{All Negatives}} = \frac{\text{TN}}{\text{TN} + \text{FN}}$$

   3. The predictive values describe the probability (0–100%) that a patient with a positive test has the disease in question and that a patient with a negative test does not have the disease in question
   4. The predictive values also describe what percentage of a population would be expected to have a disease, given a positive screening test
      a. This calculation is very important for analyzing the effects and costs of screening evaluations on asymptomatic populations

C. **If the table has more than 2 rows** of test results (e.g., answer "yes" for 0, 1, 2, 3, or 4 CAGE questions), then
   1. Sensitivity and specificity **for each row** of test results can be calculated
   2. The **predictive values** of each level of results can be calculated, as above

IV. **Diagnostics and Decision-making**

A. **Choosing the pretest probability**
   1. **For a screening test in an asymptomatic person**
      a. The pretest estimate (PTE) is the prevalence of disease in the general asymptomatic population (e.g., prevalence

of undiagnosed diabetes in the general population is about 1%; thus PTE = 0.01)

2. **For a patient with symptoms or signs**
   a. The PTE is judged by a clinician's experience or by previous studies that document the percentage of times that a symptom(s) or sign(s) may be associated with a particular disease

3. **For a patient with a test result already in hand**
   a. The PTE is the posttest probability derived from the result of the test in hand (e.g., the PTE for a pulmonary angiogram [for a possible pulmonary embolus] is the probability of an emboli as derived from the V/Q scan)

B. **Calculating the posttest probability**
   1. The **pretest estimate (PTE)** and **sensitivity (Sn)** and **specificity (Sp)** can be used to calculate the probability that a person has a disease after a positive or negative test (posttest probability) by using Bayes' theorem
   a. **If the test is positive, the posttest probability**

$$= \frac{PTE \times Sn}{(PTE \times Sn) + [(1 - PTE) \times (1 - Sp)]}$$

   i. For the purpose of multiplication, % is changed to its representative fraction between 0 and 1 (e.g., 10% = 0.1, 20% = 0.2, and so on)
   ii. **Note:** (1 – Sp) is the false positive rate
   b. **If the test is negative, then posttest probability**

$$= \frac{Sp \times (1 - PTE)}{PTE \times (1 - Sn) + [(1 - PTE) \times Sp]}$$

   i. **Note:** (1 – Sn) is the false negative rate

V. **Diagnostics: Revised**

A. Another way to the same answer is using a **nomogram**
   1. First calculate the likelihood ratios, which are the odds that a test result reflects whether a person has the disease that the test is supposed to find
   a. The **likelihood ratio for a positive test**

$$= \frac{sensitivity}{(1 - specificity)}$$

   b. The **likelihood ratio for a negative test**

$$= \frac{1 - sensitivity}{specificity}$$

   2. These ratios may be used to evaluate the accuracy at any level of test result (e.g., the 4 rows of answers generated by the CAGE questions)

B. To determine the posttest %, use a straightedge and connect the pretest % with the likelihood ratio and read the posttest percent on the righthand column

NOMOGRAM FOR INTERPRETING
DIAGNOSTIC TEST RESULTS

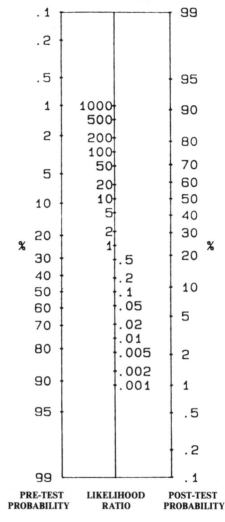

PRE-TEST PROBABILITY	LIKELIHOOD RATIO	POST-TEST PROBABILITY

EXAMPLE: Assume that in this patient the pre-test probability is 50%. Anchor a straight edge at 50% on the pre-test side of the nomogram. Assume that the likelihood ratio is 7. Direct the straight edge through the central column at 7. The post-test probability can then be read off as 8.75%. (Adapted from Fagan TJ: Nomogram for Bayes' theorem. N Engl J Med 293:257, 1975.)

VI. **Interpretation**

  A. The use of Bayes' theorem or the nomogram helps in predicting when and what test may assist in the diagnostic process

  B. The theorem or nomogram also helps in predicting when a test will not assist in the process or when using a test may produce more morbidity/mortality for false positive test results by causing diagnostic workups for false positive test results

  C. **General guidelines**

    1. **If pretest probability is very low,** then even with a test of good capability, the posttest probability may still be very low after a positive test (i.e., the probability that the test may produce a false positive may be very high)

    2. **If pretest probability is very high** (e.g., >90%), then a positive or negative test may only minimally change the posttest probability (i.e., the test may be unnecessary or may cause diagnostic confusion)

    3. Screening programs (in which prevalence is used as the pretest estimate) that use tests or evaluations of relatively excellent specificity and sensitivity (e.g., >95%) will generate—when applied to large populations—a large number of false positives and/or negatives

      a. The morbidity from the workup for all persons with positive tests may be in excess of the morbidity associated with the disease for which the test was designed to search

VII. **Summary**

  A. Choose tests carefully and consider the odds (prevalence) that an individual (group) may have the disease

  B. Indiscriminate use of tests potentially causes injury and is economically untenable

  C. In medical literature, sensitivity, specificity, and likelihood ratios are often discussed and quantified; for future reference, write down the following

    1. The specific test

    2. Exactly what the test was used for

    3. The sensitivity, specificity, and likelihood ratios or predictive values

    4. When a test is best used, as shown by the decision analysis

    5. Exceptions to the rule/analysis

    6. What alternative tests are available

  D. Use the data, along with Bayesian equation or nomogram, to help in deciding

    1. When a test may be helpful in diagnostic evaluation

    2. When a test may add confusion to diagnostic evaluation

    3. When a test is unnecessary and another test may be more effective for diagnostic evaluation

    4. When a screening test(s) for a defined population may be beneficial

References

1. Sox H: Probability theory in the use of diagnostic tests: An introduction to critical study of the literature. Ann Intern Med 104:60–66, 1986.
2. Sox H, Blatt, Higgins, Marton: Medical Decision Making. Boston, Butterworths, 1988.
3. The nomogram is from the excellent text by Sackett, Haynes, Guyatt, Tugwell: Clinical Epidemiology: A Basic Science for Clinical Epidemiology, 2nd ed. Boston, Little, Brown & Co., 1991.

Medical Literature

I. General Principles

A. When considering whether to incorporate new published information on diagnostics, prognosis, or treatment, it is important to critically evaluate the literature for
   1. Type of study
   2. Description of patients which the study evaluated
   3. Size of the population studied
   4. Clinical relevance of the study
   5. Appropriateness of the results to other subgroups
B. The incorporation of errors of judgment into standard medical care may lead, in the aggregate, to excess morbidity or mortality; for instance, the use of the cholesterol-lowering agent, clofibrate, may have resulted in up to 5,000 early deaths of asymptomatic men

II. Diagnostics as Applied to Medical Literature

A. Was the study prospective or retrospective?
B. Were the patients randomized?
C. Are characteristics of the randomized groups documented?
D. What are the eligibility/exclusion criteria?
E. What percent of eligible people were enrolled in the study?
F. What was the size of the study?
G. Were the patients drawn from a community population or were they chosen from a referral center?
H. How were the patients followed?
I. How many patients were lost to follow-up, excluded because of insufficient data, or withdrawn from the study?
J. What were the endpoints of the study and was all-cause morbidity and/or mortality included?
K. Does the study describe both placebo and active interventions?
L. Were the endpoints objectively assessed in a blinded manner?
M. Are the results statistically significant and are the test statistics (e.g., t or chi-square values) and the p values provided by the authors?

N. Are the results clinically significant?

O. Are the results applicable to the general population?

III. **Management**

A. Problems that may make the application of new protocols suspect

1. Study is not prospective, randomized, or blinded

2. Groups are not randomized properly so characteristics are dissimilar

3. There is referral bias or other selection bias

4. The eligibility/exclusion criteria are not explicit

5. Too many people were withdrawn, or lost to follow-up

   a. No more than 10–20% of group should be lost or withdrawn

   b. Patients should not be withdrawn after the study is finished

6. Patients were randomized to one group but ended up being treated in another—without a crossover-study protocol

7. The intervention or placebo is not well defined

8. The endpoints were unclear and other effects (morbidities or mortalities) were not defined

9. The statistical analysis is not well done or does not include basic statistical results (e.g., t test, probability value, confidence intervals, relative risks)

10. The study had little or no clinical relevance

B. **Successfully engineered studies/protocols may not be helpful if**

1. The study is preliminary and needs further verification on other or larger groups to detect adverse effects

2. The study has selection bias for certain subgroups (e.g., gender, age, race, comorbidities)

3. There are significant biases (e.g., referral, assessment)

C. In the final analysis, a study must be evaluated as to whether its results are applicable to your patient(s)

D. When in doubt, refer, consult and/or do further literature search

References

1. Chalmers TC, Smith H, Blackburn B, et al: A method for assessing the quality of a randomized control trial. Controlled Clin Trials 2:31–49, 1981.
2. Sackett, Haynes, Guyatt, Tugwell: Clinical Epidemiology: A Basic Science for Clinical Medicine. Boston, Little, Brown & Co., 1991.

PART VIII
APPENDICES

Appendix 1

Physical Growth Chart: Boys 2–18 Years (NCHS Percentiles)

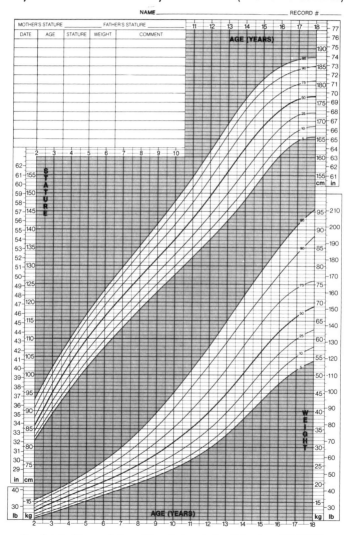

Reprinted with permission of Ross Laboratories, Columbus, OH 43216.

Physical Growth Chart: Girls 2–18 Years (NCHS Percentiles)

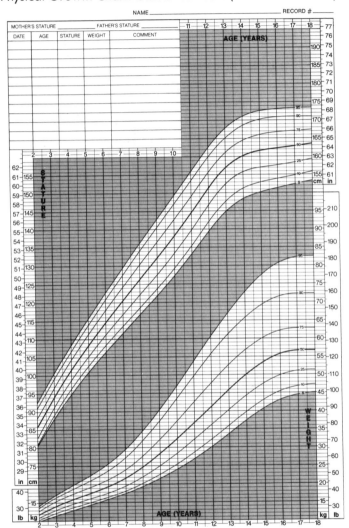

Reprinted with permission of Ross Laboratories, Columbus, OH 43216.

Appendix 2
Tanner Stages of Development

Tanner Stages of Development, Boys

Stage (Mean Age)	Genitals	Pubic Hair	Other Physical Changes
I	Testes—volume 1:5 cc; phallus—childlike	None	Preadolescent
II (11.8 years)	Testes—1.6–6.0 cc; scrotum—reddened, thinner, phallus—no change	Scarce growth of downy hair at base of penis	% body fat increases from 4.3 to 11.2
III (12.8 years)	Testes—6.0–12.cc; scrotum—greater enlargement; phallus—increased length	Pigmentation, coarsening, and curling with increased amount	Growth spurt begins in 25%
IV (13.9 years)	Testes—12.0–20.0 cc; scrotum—further enlargement and darkening; phallus—increased length and circumference	Adult pubic hair, limited area	Growth spurt begins in majority
V (14.8 years)	Testes—20.0 cc; scrotum and phallus—adult	Adult pubic hair with spread to lateral aspect thighs	Apex strength spurt

From D'Angelo LJ, Farrow J: Clinical problems in adolescent medicine. J Gen Intern Med 4:64–73, 1989, with permission. (Adapted from Tanner JM: Growth at Adolescence, 2nd ed. Oxford, Blackwell Scientific Publications, 1962.)

Tanner Stages of Development, Girls

Stage (Mean Age)	Genitals	Pubic Hair	Other Physical Changes
I	Flat, prepubertal	No true pubic hair	Preadolescent
II (10.8 years)	Small raised breast bud	Sparce growth, downy hair at sides of labia	Growth spurt begins
III (11.8 years)	General enlargement and raising of breast and areola	Pigmentation, coarsening, and curling with increased amount	Growth decelerates: 25% of girls experience menarche
IV (13.2 years)	Areola and papilla form contour separate from that of breast	Adult pubic hair, limited in area	65% of girls experience menarche
V (14.6 years)	Adult breast; areola resume same contour as breast tissue	Adult hair, classic female escutchion	10% of girls experience menarche

From D'Angelo LJ, Farrow J: Clinical problems in adolescent medicine. J Gen Intern Med 4:64–73, 1989, with permission. (Adapted from Tanner JM: Growth at Adolescence, 2nd ed. Oxford, Blackwell Scientific Publications, 1962.)

Appendix 3
Jobs at Risk

Representative Job Categories, Exposures, and Possible Diseases
to Consider When Taking an Occupational History

Job Categories	Exposures	Possible Diseases
Agricultural workers	Pesticides, infectious agents, gases, sunlight	Pesticide poisoning, farmers' lung, skin cancer
Anesthetists	Anesthetic gases	Reproductive effects, cancer
Animal handlers	Infectious agents, allergens	Asthma
Automobile workers	Asbestos, plastics, lead, solvents	Asbestosis, dermatitis
Bakers	Flour	Asthma
Battery makers	Lead, arsenic	Lead poisoning, cancer
Butchers	Vinyl plastic fumes	"Meat wrappers' asthma"
Caisson workers	Pressurized work environments	"Caisson disease," "the bends"
Carpenters	Wood dust, wood preservatives, adhesives	Nasopharyngeal cancer, dermatitis
Cement workers	Cement dust, metals	Dermatitis, bronchitis
Ceramic workers	Talc, clays	Pneumoconiosis
Demolition workers	Asbestos, wood dust	Asbestosis
Drug manufacturers	Hormones, nitroglycerin, etc.	Reproductive effects
Dry cleaners	Solvents	Liver disease, dermatitis
Dye workers	Dyestuffs, metals, solvents	Bladder cancer, dermatitis
Embalmers	Formaldehyde, infectious agents	Dermatitis
Felt makers	Mercury, polycyclic hydrocarbons	Mercuralism
Foundry workers	Silica, molten metals	Silicosis
Glass workers	Heat, solvents, metal powders	Cataracts
Hospital workers	Infectious agents, cleansers, radiation	Infections, accidents
Insulators	Asbestos, fibrous glass	Asbestosis, lung cancer, mesothelioma
Jack hammer operators	Vibration	Raynaud's phenomenon

Continued on next page.

Representative Job Categories, Exposures, and Possible Diseases
to Consider When Taking an Occupational History *(Continued)*

Job Categories	Exposures	Possible Diseases
Lathe operators	Metal dusts, cutting oils	Lung disease, cancers
Laundry workers	Bleaches, soaps, alkalis	Dermatitis
Lead burners	Lead	Lead poisoning
Miners (coal, hard rock, metals, etc.)	Talc, radiation, metals, coal dust, silica	Pneumoconioses, lung cancer
Natural gas workers	Polycyclic hydrocarbons	Lung cancer
Nuclear workers	Radiation, plutonium	Metal poisoning, cancer
Office workers	Poor lighting, poorly designed equipment	Joint problems, eye problems
Painters	Paints, solvents, spackling compounds	Neurologic problems
Paper makers	Acids, alkalis, solvents, metals	Lung disorders, dermatitis
Petroleum workers	Polycyclic hydrocarbons, catalysts, zeolites	Cancer, pneumoconiosis
Plumbers	Lead, solvents, asbestos	Lead poisoning
Railroad workers	Creosote, sunlight, oils, solvents	Cancer, dermatitis
Seamen	Sunlight, asbestos	Cancer, accidents
Smelter workers	Metals, heat, sulfur dioxide, arsenic	Cancer
Steel workers	Heat, metals, silica	Cataracts, heat stroke
Stone cutters	Silica	Silicosis
Textile workers	Cotton dust, fabrics, finishers, dyes, carbon disulfide	Bysinossis, dermatitis, psychosis
Varnish makers	Solvents, waxes	Dermatitis
Vineyard workers	Arsenic, pesticides	Cancer, dermatitis
Welders	Fumes, nonionizing radiation	Lead poisoning, cataracts

From Rom WN (ed): Environmental and Occupational Medicine. Boston, Little, Brown and Co., 1983, with permission.

Occupational Diseases of the Respiratory Tract

Type	Examples of Associated Exposure
Acute or Recurrent	
Upper respiratory inflammation	Fibrous glass, metal dust, welding, and plastic fumes
Airway disorders	
Asthma	Western red cedar, toluene diisocyanate
Airway irritation, including nonspecific hyperreactivity	Welding fumes, irritant gases
Byssinosis	Cotton and flax processing
Extrinsic allergic alveolitis	Wood dust, thermophilic actinomycetes
Toxic pneumonitis	Cadmium, oxides of nitrogen
Pleural effusion	Asbestos
Chronic	
Interstitial diseases (pneumoconioses)	Silicates, coal dust
Granulomatous disease	Beryllium
Chronic bronchitis	Metal dusts, coal dust
Chronic pleural diseases	
Pleural thickening and rounded atelectasis	Asbestos
Diffuse malignant mesothelioma	Asbestos
Carcinoma	
Upper respiratory tract	Chromium, nickel, hardwood dust
Bronchogenic	Coal tar pitch volatiles, asbestos, arsenic

Reprinted with permission from the American College of Physicians.

Occupational Disorders of the Kidney and Bladder

Condition	Class of Associated Exposures	Example(s) of Specific Agents
Acute renal disease		
Tubulointerstitial	Halogenated hydrocarbons	Carbon tetrachloride
	Pesticides	Parathion, DDT*
	Heavy metals	Arsenic, mercury, lead
Tubulointerstitial (indirect injury)	Hemolytic agents	Arsine
	Rhabdomyolytic agents	Ethylene glycol, cresol
	Physical stress	Heat
Glomerular	Organic solvents	Styrene
	Heavy metals	Lead, mercury
Chronic renal disease		
Tubulointerstitial	Heavy metals	Cadmium, lead
Glomerular	Heavy metals	Lead, mercury
	Organic solvents	Styrene
Bladder disease		
Bladder dysfunction (sacral neuropathy)	Plasticizer	Dimethylaminopropionitrile
Bladder carcinoma	Dyes	Benzidine

* DDT = dichlorodiphenyltrichloroethane.
Reprinted with permission from the American College of Physici ‑‑

Gastrointestinal Symptoms and Occupational Exposures

Symptom	Type of Exposures	Example
Nausea and vomiting	Organic solvents	Acetone, benzene
	Cholinesterase inhibitors	Carbaryl, malathion
	Methemoglobin formers	Nitrotoluene
	Irritants	Epoxy, resins, copper fumes
	Asphyxiants	Carbon monoxide
Constipation	Metals	Lead, thallium
Diarrhea	Infectious agents	Leptospirosis
	Cholinesterase inhibitors	Malathion
	Metals	Arsenic

Reprinted with permission from the American College of Physicians.

Occupationally Related Liver Disease

Type	Agent Class	Examples
Acute		
Acute hepatocellular disease	Chlorinated hydrocarbons*	Trichloroethylene
	Chlorinated aromatics	Polychlorinated biphenyls
	Organic amines	Nitrosamine
	Nitro(so) compounds	Trinotrotoluene
	Ethers	Dioxane
	Aromatic/aliphatic hydrocarbons*	White spirit
	Inorganic	Phosphorus
	Virus*	Hepatitis A; B; non-A, non-B
Acute cholestatic hepatitis	Epoxy resin	Methylpredianiline
Chronic		
Hepatoportal sclerosis	Metals	Arsenicals
Chronic persistent hepatocellular disease	Chlorinated aromatics	Polychlorinated biphenyls
Granulomatous hepatitis	Metals	Beryllium
Cirrhosis	Metals	Arsenicals
	Haloalkenes	Vinyl chloride
	Chlorinated hydrocarbons (?)	Carbon tetrachloride
Angiosarcoma	Metals	Thorium dioxide
	Haloalkenes	Vinyl chloride
Hepatoma	Metals	Arsenicals
	Haloalkenes	Vinyl chloride
	Chlorinated hydrocarbons (?)	Trichloroethylene

* Also associated with subacute hepatocellular disease.
Reprinted with permission from the American College of Physicians.

Appendix 4
Occupational History Form

I. **Work and Exposure History**

    A. *Current Employment*

        Questions 1–7 refer to your current or most recent job.

        1. Job title _____

        2. Type of industry _____

        3. Name of employer _____

        4. Year job began _____

           Still working?

           Yes _____ No _____ If no, year job ended _____

        5. Briefly desribe this job, noting any part that you feel may be hazardous to your health.

        _____

        _____

        6. Do you wear protective equipment on this job?

           Yes _____ No _____ If yes, check equipment used:

           Gloves _____   Air supply respirator _____

           Mask respirator _____   Coveralls or apron _____

           Hearing protection _____   Safety glasses _____

        7. In this job, are you exposed to any of the following?

           If yes, mark those to which you are exposed:

           Fumes and dusts _____   Elements and metals _____

           Solvents _____   Other chemicals _____   Noise _____

           Vibration _____   Excess heat/cold _____

           Emotional stress _____   Other _____

    B. *Employment History*

        It is important that we know all the jobs you have had. Job #1 is your current or most recent job. Beginning with the job before this one—Job #2—please fill in as much of the information requested as you can remember, and continue to do so until all previous jobs have been listed. Include any military service you have had. If need additional space, use the back of this form.

	YEARS From–To	JOB TITLE	EXPOSURES
Job #2	_____	_____	_____
Job #3	_____	_____	_____
Job #4	_____	_____	_____
Job #5	_____	_____	_____
Job #6	_____	_____	_____
Job #7	_____	_____	_____
Job #8	_____	_____	_____
Wartime employment	_____	_____	_____

    C. *Other Exposures*

        1. Does anyone in your household work at a job that you suspect involves exposures that may be brought home from work (e.g., asbestos fibers on clothes)?

           Yes _____ No _____

2. Are there any industries in the area in which you live that may pollute your environment?
Yes ＿＿＿ No ＿＿＿

3. Do you have any hobbies that expose you to chemicals, metals, or other substances?
Yes ＿＿＿ No ＿＿＿

4. Have you ever smoked cigarettes? ("No" means less than 20 packs of cigarettes in your entire life.) Yes ＿＿＿ No ＿＿＿
If yes, please answer the following:
   a. Do you now smoke cigarettes (that is, as of 1 month ago)?
   Yes ＿＿＿ No ＿＿＿
   b. How many years have you smoked? ＿＿＿
   c. Of the entire time you have smoked, about how many cigarettes per day do or did you smoke on the average ＿＿＿

II. General Health History

1. Is there any particular hazard or part of your job that you think relates to your problem?
Yes ＿＿＿ No ＿＿＿

2. Do any of your coworkers have problems or complaints similar to yours?
Yes ＿＿＿ No ＿＿＿

---

* For each positive response to review of systems, ask whether symptoms are better, worse, or no different in associaton with work.

From Rosenstock L, Cullen MR: Clinical Occupational Medicine. Philadelphia, WB Saunders, 1986, with permission.

Appendix 5
Mini-Mental State Examination

Patient's Name _____
Date Administered _____

Maximum Score	Patient Score	
		Orientation
5	____	What is the (year) (season) (date) (day) (month)?
5	____	Where are we: (state) (country) (town) (hospital) (floor)?
		Registration
3	____	Name three objects—1 second to say each. Then ask the patient all three after you have said them.
		Give one point for each correct answer. Then repeat them until patient learns all three. Count trials and record.
		Number of Trials ____
		Attention and Calculation
5	____	Serial sevens. One point for each correct. Stop after five answers. If subject refuses, spell "WORLD" backwards.
		Recall
3	____	Ask for three objects repeated above. Give one point for each correct.
		Language
9	____	Name a pencil and watch. (2 points)
		Repeat the following: "No ifs, ands, or buts." (1 point)
		Follow a three-stage command: "Take a paper in your right hand, fold it in half, and put it on the floor." (3 points)
		Read and obey the following: "Close your eyes." (1 point)
		Write a sentence. (1 point)
		Copy design. (1 point)

30	____	
Maximum Score	Patient Total	

ASSESS level of consciousness along a continuum.

Alert	Drowsy	Stupor	Coma

From Hazzard W, et al: Principles of Geriatric Medicine and Gerontology, 2nd ed. New York, McGraw Hill, Inc., 1990, with permission.

Appendix 6
Useful Equations

I. Renal
   A. Estimated creatinine clearance

      1. For men = $\dfrac{(140 - age) \times (wt\ in\ kg)}{72 \times serum\ creatinine\ (mg/dl)}$

      2. For women =   (same equation) × 0.85

   B. Fractional excretions

      1. FeNa = $\dfrac{U(Na) \times P(Cr)}{P(Na) \times U(Cr)} \times 100$

         a. FeNa: $<$ 1 = prerenal
         b. FeNa: $>$ 1 = renal (ATN)

      2. FeU = $\dfrac{U(u) \times P(Cr)}{BUN \times U(Cr)} \times 100$

         a. FeU: $<$ 0.3 = prerenal
         b. FeU: 0.4–0.7 = renal (ATN)

   C. Anion gap (normal = 8–12 mEq)
      1. **Note:** the "normal" range is laboratory-dependent
      2. = Na – (Cl + Bicarb)

   D. Osmolar concentrations (normal = 290 mOsm/kg2.H_2O)
      1. = 2 × (Na) + blood glucose/18 + BUN/2.8
         a. If patient inebriated, add ETOH level/3.4
      2. Osmolal gap (normal $<$ 10 mOsm/kg.H_2O)

   E. Total body water (TBW)
      1. Men =   0.6 × lean body weight
      2. Women = 0.5 × lean body weight

II. Respiratory
   A. Aa gradient (normal = 3–16 mmHg)
      1. = $PO_2 - PaO_2 = PO_2 - [(FIO_2 \times 713) - PaCO_2/0.8]$
      2. To correct for age, add (2.5 + 0.25 × [age]) to the computation above

Appendix 7
Cutaneous Innervation*

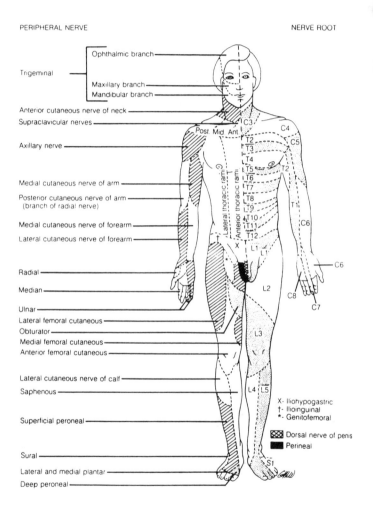

PERIPHERAL NERVE   NERVE ROOT

Trigeminal
- Ophthalmic branch
- Maxillary branch
- Mandibular branch

Anterior cutaneous nerve of neck
Supraclavicular nerves
Axillary nerve
Medial cutaneous nerve of arm
Posterior cutaneous nerve of arm (branch of radial nerve)
Medial cutaneous nerve of forearm
Lateral cutaneous nerve of forearm
Radial
Median
Ulnar
Lateral femoral cutaneous
Obturator
Medial femoral cutaneous
Anterior femoral cutaneous
Lateral cutaneous nerve of calf
Saphenous
Superficial peroneal
Sural
Lateral and medial plantar
Deep peroneal

X- Iliohypogastric
†- Ilioinguinal
*- Genitofemoral

Dorsal nerve of penis
Perineal

* The segmental or radicular (root) distribution is shown on the left side of the body and the peripheral nerve distribution on the right side of the body.

From Simon RP, Aminoff MJ, Greenberg DA: Clinical Neurology. Norwalk, CT, Appleton & Lange, 1989, pp 164–165, with permission.

NERVE ROOT   PERIPHERAL NERVE

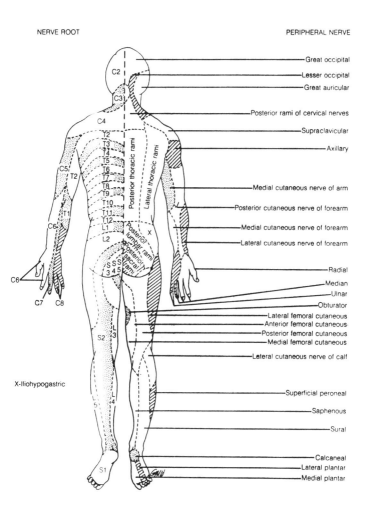

X-Iliohypogastric

PART IX
INDEX OF CONSENSUSES

Agency for Health Care Policy and Research (AHCPR)

Urinary Incontinence Guideline Panel: Urinary Incontinence in Adults: Quick Reference Guide for Clinicians. AHCPR Publication Nos. 92-0038, 92-0041. Rockville, MD, Agency for Health Care Policy and Research, March 1992.

American Academy of Dermatology (AAD)

Guidelines of care for acne vulgaris. J Am Acad Dermatol 22(April):676–680, 1990.

American Academy of Ophthalmology (AAO)

Cataract in the otherwise healthy adult eye. San Francisco, American Academy of Ophthalmology, January 1990.

Screening guidelines for diabetic retinopathy. Ann Intern Med 116(April): 683–685, 1992 (in collaboration with American College of Physicians and American Diabetic Association).

American Board of Internal Medicine (ABIM)

Attributes of the general internist and recommendations for training. Am Rev Respir Dis 134:371, 1986.

American Cancer Society (ACS)

Summary of current guidelines for the cancer-related checkup. In American Cancer Society Textbook of Clinical Oncology. Atlanta, American Cancer Society, 1991.

American College of Obstetrics and Gynecology (ACOG)

Amenorrhea. ACOG Technical Bulletin No. 128, Washington, DC, May 1989.

Carcinoma of the Breast. ACOG Technical Bulletin No. 158, Washington, DC, August 1991.

Estrogen Replacement Therapy. ACOG Technical Bulletin No. 93, June 1986.

Nonmalignant Conditions of the Breast. ACOG Technical Bulletin No. 156, June 1991.

Oral Contraception. ACOG Technical Bulletin No. 106, July 1987.

Osteoporosis. ACOG Technical Bulletin No. 118, July 1988.

American College of Physicians (ACP)

The American College of Physicians Ethics Manual. Part 1: History; The Patient; Other Physicians. Ann Intern Med 111(August):245–252, 1989.

The American College of Physicians Ethics Manual. Part 2: The Physician and Society; Research; Life-Sustaining Treatment; Other Issues. Ann Intern Med 111(August):327–335, 1989.

Chemical Dependence. Philadelphia, American College of Physicians. September 14, 1984.

Disulfiram treatment of alcoholism. Ann Intern Med 111(December):943–945, 1989.

Eating disorders: Anorexia and bulimia. Ann Intern Med 105(November):790–794, 1986.

Endoscopy in the evaluation of dyspepsia. Ann Intern Med 102(February):266–269, 1985.

Health care needs of the adolescent. Ann Intern Med. 110(June):930–935, 1989.

How to study the gallbladder. Ann Intern Med 109(November):752–754, 1988.

Indications for carotid endarterectomy. Ann Intern Med 111(October):675–677, 1989.

Methods for stopping cigarette smoking. Ann Intern Med 105(August): 281–291, 1986.

The use of diagnostic tests for screening and evaluating breast lesions. Ann Intern Med 103(July):147–151, 1985.

Occupational and environmental medicine: The internist's role. Ann Intern Med 113(December):974–982, 1990.

Practice strategies for elective red blood transfusion. Ann Intern Med 116(March):403–406, 1992.

Preoperative pulmonary function testing. Ann Intern Med 112(May):793–794, 1990.

Selected methods for the management of diabetes mellitus. Ann Intern Med 99(August):272–274, 1983.

American College of Radiology (ACR)

On Sonography for the Detection and Diagnosis of Breast Disease. Reston, VA, ACR, September 1984.

Guidelines for Mammography. ACR, September 1992.

American College of Rheumatology (formerly the American Rheumatism Association)

Dictionary of the Rheumatic Diseases: Volume I and II. American Rheumatism Association, 1985.

Guidelines for Reviewers of Rheumatic Disease Care. American College of Rheumatology, 1989.

American Diabetes Association

Diabetes mellitus and exercise. Diabetes Care 13(July):785–789, 1990. Reprinted 14(Suppl 2):52–56, 1991.

Diabetic neuropathy. Diabetes Care 14(Suppl 2):63–68, March 1991.

Foot care in patients with diabetes mellitus. Diabetes Care 14(Suppl 2):18–19, March 1991.

Hospital admission guidelines for diabetes mellitus. Diabetes Care 13(November):1118–1119, 1990.

Office guide to diagnosis and classification of diabetes mellitus and other categories of glucose intolerance. Diabetes care 14(Suppl 2):3–4, March 1991.

Screening for diabetes. Diabetes Care 12:588–590, 1989. Reprinted 14(Suppl 2): 7–9, 1991.

Screening guidelines for diabetic retinopathy. Ann Intern Med 116(April):683–685, 1992 (in conjunction with the American College of Physicians and the American Academy of Ophthalmology).

Standards of medical care for patients with diabetes. Diabetes Care 12(May):365–368, 1989.

American Gastroenterological Association (AGA)

Clinical evaluation of jaundice. JAMA 262:3031–3034, 1989.

Detection and surveillance of colorectal cancer. JAMA 261(January):580–585, 1989.

American Heart Association (AHA)

Prevention of bacterial endocarditis. JAMA 264(December):1919–1922, 1990.

Guidelines for the diagnosis of rheumatic fever, Jones criteria, 1992 update. JAMA 268(October):2069–2073, 1992.

Jones criteria (revised) for guidance in the diagnosis of rheumatic fever. Circulation 69:204A, 1984.

American Medical Association (AMA)

HIV Early Care: AMA Physician Guidelines. Chicago, AMA, 1991.

American Thoracic Society (ATS)

Prevention of influenza and pneumonia. Am Rev Respir Dis 142:487–488, 1990.

Treatment of tuberculosis and tuberculosis infection in adults and children. Am Rev Respir Dis 134:355–362, 1986.

The diagnosis of nonmalignant disease related to asbestos. Am Rev Respir Dis 134:363–368, 1986.

Standards for the diagnosis and care of patients with chronic obstructive pulmonary disease (COPD) and asthma. Am Rev Respir Dis 136:225–243, 1987.

American Thyroid Association (ATA)

Guidelines for the use of laboratory tests in thyroid disorders. JAMA 263:1529–1532, 1990.

American Urological Association (AUA)

Guidelines for Urologic Care. Baltimore, AUA, February 1987.

Centers for Disease Control (CDC)

Pelvic inflammatory disease: Guidelines for prevention and management. MMWR 40(RR-5):1–25, April 1991.

Prevention and control of influenza. Ann Intern Med 107(October):521–525, 1987.

The Prevention and Treatment of Complications of Diabetes Mellitus: A Guide for Primary Care Physicians. Atlanta, CDC, 1991.

Recommendations for diagnosing and treating syphilis in HIV-infected patients. MMWR 37(29):601–608, October 1988.

Recommendations for prophylaxis against *Pneumocystis carinii* pneumonia for adults and adolescents infected with human immunodeficiency virus. MMWR 41(RR-4): April 1992.

Screening for tuberculosis and tuberculosis infection in high-risk populations. MMWR 39:1–12, May 1990.

Sexually transmitted diseases treatment guidelines: 1989. MMWR 38(S-8):5–15, September 1989.

Update on adult immunization. MMWR 40(RR-12): November 1991.

The use of preventive therapy for tuberculosis infection in the United States. MMWR 39(RR-8):9–12, May 1990.

National Institutes of Health

Detection, evaluation, and treatment of renovascular hypertension. Arch Intern Med 147(May):820–829, 1987.

Differential diagnosis of dementing diseases. JAMA 258:3411–3416, 1987.

Gastrointestinal infections in AIDS. Ann Intern Med 116:63–77, 1992.

Guidelines for the Diagnosis and Management of Asthma. Bethesda, MD, NIH Publication No. 91-304A, June 1991.

Prophylaxis and treatment of osteoporosis. Am J Med 90(January):107–110, 1991.

Rand Corporation

United States Preventive Services Task Force (USPSTF)

INDEX